Day-to-day Challenges in Facial Plastic Surgery

Editor

WILLIAM H. TRUSWELL

FACIAL PLASTIC SURGERY CLINICS OF NORTH AMERICA

www.facialplastic.theclinics.com

Consulting Editor
J. REGAN THOMAS

November 2020 • Volume 28 • Number 4

ELSEVIER

1600 John F. Kennedy Boulevard • Suite 1800 • Philadelphia, Pennsylvania, 19103-2899

http://www.theclinics.com

FACIAL PLASTIC SURGERY CLINICS OF NORTH AMERICA Volume 28, Number 4
November 2020 ISSN 1064-7406, ISBN-13: 978-0-323-69816-0

Editor: Stacy Eastman
Developmental Editor: Julia McKenzie

Facial Plastic Surgery Clinics of North America (ISSN 1064-7406) is published quarterly by Elsevier Inc., 360 Park Avenue South, New York, NY 10010-1710. Months of issue are February, May, August, and November. Business and Editorial Offices: 1600 John F. Kennedy Blvd., Suite 1800, Philadelphia, PA 19103-2899. Periodicals postage paid at New York, NY, and additional mailing offices. Subscription prices are $408.00 per year (US individuals), $692.00 per year (US institutions), $454.00 per year (Canadian individuals), $861.00 per year (Canadian institutions), $535.00 per year (foreign individuals), $861.00 per year (foreign institutions), $100.00 per year (US students), $100.00 per year (Canadian students), and $255.00 per year (foreign students). Foreign air speed delivery is included in all *Clinics* subscription prices. All prices are subject to change without notice. POSTMASTER: Send address changes to *Facial Plastic Surgery Clinics*, Elsevier Health Sciences Division, Subscription Customer Service, 3251 Riverport Lane, Maryland Heights, MO 63043. **Customer service: 1-800-654-2452 (US and Canada); 1-314-447-8871 (outside US and Canada); Fax: 314-447-8029; E-mail: journalscustomerservice-usa@elsevier.com (for print support); journalsonlinesupport-usa@elsevier.com (for online support).**

Reprints. For copies of 100 or more of articles in this publication, please contact the Commercial Reprints Department, Elsevier Inc., 360 Park Avenue South, New York, NY 10010-1710. Tel.: 212-633-3874; Fax: 212-633-3820; E-mail: reprints@elsevier.com.

Facial Plastic Surgery Clinics of North America is covered in *MEDLINE/PubMed* (*Index Medicus*).

Contributors

CONSULTING EDITOR

J. REGAN THOMAS, MD
Professor, Facial Plastic and Reconstructive
Surgery, Department of Otolaryngology–Head
and Neck Surgery, Northwestern University
Feinberg School of Medicine, Chicago, Illinois,
USA

EDITOR

WILLIAM H. TRUSWELL IV, MD, FACS
President, American Board of Facial Plastic
and Reconstructive Surgery, Past President,
American Academy of Facial Plastic and
Reconstructive Surgery, Private Practice,
Easthampton, Massachusetts, USA

AUTHORS

**PETER A. ADAMSON, OONT, MD, FRCS,
FACS**
Professor, Division of Facial Plastic and
Reconstructive Surgery, Department of
Otolaryngology–Head and Neck Surgery,
University of Toronto Faculty of Medicine,
Toronto, Ontario, Canada

ROXANA COBO, MD
Coordinator, Service of Otolaryngology, Centro
Médico Imbanaco, Cali, Colombia

MARK CONSTANTIAN, MD, FACS
Plastic and Reconstructive Surgeon, Division
of Plastic Surgery, Department of Surgery,
University of Wisconsin School of Medicine
and Public Health, Madison, Wisconsin, USA;
Department of Surgery, University of Virginia
Medical School, Charlottesville, Virginia, USA

STEVEN H. DAYAN, MD, FACS
Division of Facial Plastic and Reconstructive
Surgery, Department of Otolaryngology,
Chicago Center for Facial Plastic Surgery,
University of Illinois at Chicago, Chicago,
Illinois, USA

AMANDA E. DILGER, MD
AAFPRS Fellow, Facial Plastic and
Reconstructive Surgery, Beverly Hills,
California, USA; Roseville Facial
Plastic Surgery, Roseville, California,
USA

FRED G. FEDOK, MD, FACS
Adjunct Professor, Department of Surgery,
University of South Alabama Mobile,
Fedok Plastic Surgery, Foley, Alabama,
USA

RICHARD D. GENTILE, MD, MBA
Medical Director, Facial Plastic Surgery,
Gentile Facial Plastic Surgery & Aesthetic Laser
Center, Youngstown, Ohio, USA; Staff
Physician, Facial Plastic Surgery, Cleveland
Clinic Akron General Hospital, Akron, Ohio,
USA

MARK M. HAMILTON, MD, FACS
Assistant Clinical Professor of Otolaryngology–
Head and Neck Surgery, Indiana University
School of Medicine, Indianapolis, Indiana,
USA

THUY-VAN T. HO, MD
Rejuvenation Medical Aesthetics, Newtown, Pennsylvania, USA

ARI HYMAN, MD
Private Practice, Facial Plastic and Reconstructive Surgery, Encino, California, USA

RICHARD KAO, MD
Resident, Department of Otolaryngology–Head and Neck Surgery, Indiana University School of Medicine, Indianapolis, Indiana, USA

SAMUEL M. LAM, MD, FACS, FISHRS
Private Practice, Lam Facial Plastics, Plano, Texas, USA

PHILLIP R. LANGSDON, MD
The Langsdon Clinic, Germantown, Tennessee, USA; Department of Otolaryngology–Head and Neck Surgery, Professor, Chief of Facial Plastic Surgery, University of Tennessee Health Science Center, Memphis, Tennessee, USA

JESSYKA G. LIGHTHALL, MD
Director, Facial Plastic & Reconstructive Surgery, Associate Professor, Department of Otolaryngology–Head & Neck Surgery, Penn State College of Medicine, Hershey, Pennsylvania, USA

JOHN RHEE, MD, MPH
Professor & Chair, Department of Otolaryngology Head and Neck Surgery, Medical College of Wisconsin, Milwaukee, Wisconsin, USA

JORDAN RIHANI, MD, FACS
Facial Plastic Surgery Institute, Southlake, Texas, USA

RONALD J. SCHROEDER II, MD
Midwest Facial Plastic Surgery, Woodbury, Minnesota, USA

JONATHAN M. SYKES, MD
Professor Emeritus, Facial Plastic Surgery, UC Davis Medical Center, Sacramento, California, USA; Director, Facial Plastic Surgery, Roxbury Institute, Beverly Hills, California, USA

SHERARD AUSTIN TATUM III, MD, FAAP, FACS
Professor of Otolaryngology and Pediatrics, Interim Chair, Department of Otolaryngology, Medical Director, Cleft and Craniofacial Center, Division of Facial Plastic and Reconstructive Surgery, Upstate Medical University, State University of New York, Syracuse, New York, USA

WILLIAM H. TRUSWELL, MD, FACS
President, American Board of Facial Plastic and Reconstructive Surgery, Past President, American Academy of Facial Plastic and Reconstructive Surgery, Private Practice, Easthampton, Massachusetts, USA

ANA MARIA ELISABETH (ANITA) WEVER, MSc
Clinical Psychologist, Almere, The Netherlands

CASPER CANDIDO (CAPI) WEVER, MD, PhD
Facial Plastic Surgeon, Department of Otolaryngology, Head & Neck Surgery, Leiden University Medical Center, Leiden, The Netherlands

CATHERINE WINSLOW, MD
Assistant Clinical Professor, IU School of Medicine, Owner, Winslow Facial Plastic Surgery, Carmel, Indiana, USA

Contents

> Facial plastic surgeons need to be very much more than excellent surgeons. They need to understand and have the ability to bring each patient into the practice family of the surgeon, the administrative and clerical staff, the nurses, the technicians, and the aestheticians. The entire staff must "own" the practice and the patient management philosophy of the surgeon. This article is the author's philosophy and method of guiding his patients through their journey of rejuvenative facial surgery based on 44 years of experience.

> The facial plastic surgeon faces increasing competition in the aesthetic world for both surgical and nonsurgical services. Incorporating nonsurgical options in practice, such as "liquid facelifts," aesthetic services, and products, increases both patient satisfaction and office revenue stream. A successful nonsurgical practice can be built with minimal expense by focusing on the most critical and popular options to offer patients.

> In this article the authors discuss and analyze technological devices also known as energy-based devices and their use in skin rejuvenation, facial contouring, skin tightening, and other applications in facial plastic surgery. Energy has been applied in some form to tissue since the beginning of recorded history. The practice of applying heat to tissue with the use of cauters was used for thousands of years as an invaluable method of controlling hemorrhage. Continuous improvement of methods for using the beneficial effects of heat on tissue eventually led to the development of the basic concepts of electrosurgery we know today.

> Body dysmorphic disorder and borderline personality disorder are common in esthetic practices and occur in up to 15% of patients. Operating on these patients

may not only lead to dissatisfaction but may also worsen their premorbid condition and can induce negative behavior toward the practice. Preventing surgery and referring patients for cognitive therapy is essential. An adequate understanding of these conditions and the available screening tools is indispensable for all esthetic practitioners. Unrealistic emotional attribution to a facial shape, multiple procedures, a near-normal nose at the outset, childhood trauma, multiple comorbid mental conditions, and social dysfunction are red-flags to consider.

Patient satisfaction is the ultimate measure of success in cosmetic facial plastic surgery. A successful outcome depends on patient selection, technical performance, and postoperative care. Patient perception can be influenced by physician–patient interactions. Surgical training focuses on diagnosis—identifying variations in physical condition and treatment. Although these skills are essential to a well-trained and successful facial plastic surgeon, the importance of proper patient selection, management of expectations, and empathetic communication in cosmetic surgery are often overlooked in education and cannot be understated. This article outlines the contributing factors to difficult physician–patient relationships and strategies for mitigating these situations.

Surgical education is under tremendous pressure due to ever-increasing medical knowledge and demands on trainees' time. They must continually learn more in less time due to work hour limitations, regulations, and electronic medical record demands. Surgical training must become more efficient. There is an unprecedented array of education and training opportunities for resident preparation. The preparation for each case has to be maximal. Preoperative, intraoperative, and postoperative simulation and discussions improve the educational benefit of the trainee experience. For the teaching surgeon, putting a scalpel in residents' hands requires patience, knowledge, judgment, and a leap of faith in the resident.

This article seeks to inform facial plastic surgeons about the evolving issues that affect contemporary medical literature and the publishing landscape. We hope to shed light on the key metrics that influence a journal's decision to accept a particular submission and how these metrics are predicated on a rapidly changing landscape within the academic and public community. The key metrics are: citations, number of views, and social media or public attention. These metrics produce what we call "high impact" articles. This article introduces bibliometric terms and further defines the metrics that are most important to a journal.

Complications in facial plastic surgery can occur in both surgical and nonsurgical procedures. Many complications can be prevented through thorough preprocedural evaluation, patient counseling, and close postoperative monitoring. Despite the best efforts complications will happen and identifying them early is critical to prevent long-term sequelae. It is important to know how to both manage the complication and guide the patient through the recovery process.

Skin resurfacing techniques allow improvement of skin texture and color. This includes the effacement of wrinkles, signs of photoaging, and the softening of scars. Laser resurfacing, chemical peels, and dermabrasion are associated with overlapping risks of complications. The most common of these include infection, hypopigmentation, hyperpigmentation, and scarring. Patient evaluation helps provide treatment that gives the maximal benefit with a minimization of risks. This includes understanding the extent of each patient's issues (Glogau scale) and Fitzpatrick type. A thorough knowledge of potential risks will reduce their incidence and optimize early recognition and treatment of these complications when they do occur.

Facial plastic surgery has thrived in both academic and private settings. In this article, 3 surgeons comment on a variety of selected topics that are pertinent to their lives as academic and private practice surgeons.

Social media has become a rising popular online medium for facilitating the exchange of information and ideas for the purpose of education and networking, especially in the realm of plastic surgeon. It is important for facial plastic surgeons in private practice to recognize the influence of and engagement in social media, particularly among younger adults given the ongoing movement of cosmetic patients seeking facial rejuvenation treatments at an earlier age. This article discusses the most recent trends in social media and facial plastic surgery as well as the benefits and challenges of social media in private practice.

This article offers a practical approach for cosmetic surgeons to develop and enhance their clinical practice by offering pearls that have worked for the author. Leadership of staff is the cornerstone of developing a successful business practice by hiring, retaining, and inspiring key talent. It is important to develop a clear vision for a practice and to articulate a unique selling proposition that can attract patients and be effectively communicated by authentic videos. Peers can be a source of accountability and feedback and can help provide support and structure to a business owner.

Understanding and Getting Involved in the International Facial Plastic Surgery Community

Roxana Cobo and Peter A. Adamson

This article is intended to engage international facial plastic and reconstructive surgeons so they can maximally benefit from the increased connectivity fostered by the Internet. Facial plastic surgeons are encouraged to participate in the educational programs being developed by the International Federation of Facial Plastic Surgery Societies. Many international surgeons grapple with the issues surrounding the development or expansion of their own facial plastic and reconstructive surgery practices. The Strategy Circle and suggestions on how to acquire knowledge and surgical skills are discussed. Practical recommendations to assist in transitioning a practice to facial plastic and reconstructive surgery are provided.

FACIAL PLASTIC SURGERY CLINICS OF NORTH AMERICA

SERIES OF RELATED INTEREST

Clinics in Plastic Surgery
https://www.plasticsurgery.theclinics.com
Otolaryngologic Clinics
https://www.oto.theclinics.com
Dermatologic Clinics
https://www.derm.theclinics.com

THE CLINICS ARE AVAILABLE ONLINE!
Access your subscription at:
www.theclinics.com

Foreword
Day-to-Day Challenges in Facial Plastic Surgery

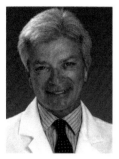

J. Regan Thomas, MD
Consulting Editor

This issue of *Facial Plastic Surgery Clinics of North America* addresses unique but important and very practical issues that confront facial plastic surgeons practicing in today's contemporary environment. A useful range of pragmatic articles presenting suggestions for dealing with a variety of challenges facing todays practitioners is presented.

Facial plastic surgery practice is now impacted and influenced by factors that were not issues even a few years ago, issues, such as social media, office based nonsurgical facial and aesthetic skin treatment modalities, and business practice management options and opportunities that must be addressed by todays specialists. The *Facial Plastic Surgery Clinics of North America* is pleased to provide insight and suggestions for these challenges and necessities in contemporary facial plastic practice.

Dr William Truswell as guest editor has developed a variety of articles addressing these practical practice issues. He has assembled an experienced and expert group of contributing authors to share their insights on aspects of modern practice. In addition to practice management and modern procedure applications being explored, patient interaction issues are also discussed. These include dealing with the unhappy patient, patients with complications of treatment, and patients with various personality disorders.

I am confident that this unique issue will prove to be extremely useful and of real-world usefulness to our readers. Dr Truswell and his experienced expert contributing authors have accomplished an important reference for today's facial plastic surgery practice environment.

J. Regan Thomas, MD
Facial Plastic and Reconstructive Surgery
Department of Otolaryngology
Head and Neck Surgery
Northwestern University of Medicine
675 North Saint Clair Street
Suite 15-200
Chicago, IL 60611, USA

E-mail address:
Regan.Thomas@nm.org

Facial Plast Surg Clin N Am 28 (2020) xi
https://doi.org/10.1016/j.fsc.2020.08.001
1064-7406/20/© 2020 Published by Elsevier Inc.

Preface

Day-to-Day Challenges in Facial Plastic Surgery

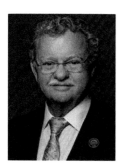

William H. Truswell IV, MD, FACS
Editor

Facial plastic and reconstructive surgeons' professional lives are first consumed with starting a practice, academic or private, building the practice, and being facial plastic surgeons. We live our lives as experts in our chosen field. However, there are many issues that arise sometimes suddenly to startle us, other times lingering in the background waiting for attention. The articles in this issue of the *Facial Plastic Surgery Clinics of North America* explore many day-to-day problems that are often overlooked, seldom formerly taught, but present challenges to the smooth running of our practices. The advice herein explores ways to guide patients through the journey of rejuvenation, how to incorporate nonsurgical and cosmetic options into a surgical practice, and the way to decide how to purchase wisely and utilize high tech equipment in an aesthetic setting. One article advises how to recognize and deal with patients with personality disorders, and another discusses how to handle angry and unhappy patients. One article explores balancing academic duties and a busy cosmetic surgery practice. Another reflects on the challenge of teaching residents to become

surgeons and allowing them to pick up the scalpel. A third article looks at the comparison of a full-time academic practice vis-a-vis a private solo practice. Complications of procedures are issues that we constantly are on the lookout for and guard against. Two articles explore this: one on complications of surgery and the other of resurfacing techniques. Getting published, something many wish to do but find it hard to get started, is the topic of another article. On the business side of practice, there is a discussion on leveraging social media and another on good business moves to enhance your practice. Last, understanding and getting involved in the international facial plastic community are investigated.

William H. Truswell IV, MD, FACS
Private Practice
123 Union Street, Suite 100
Easthampton, MA 01027, USA

E-mail address:
bill.truswell@gmail.com

Facial Plast Surg Clin N Am 28 (2020) xiii
https://doi.org/10.1016/j.fsc.2020.08.002
1064-7406/20/© 2020 Published by Elsevier Inc.

From "Hello to Goodbye"— Guiding the Patient of Her Journey Through Facial Rejuvenation Surgery

William H. Truswell, MD[a,b,c,d],*

KEYWORDS

- Facelift • Consultation • Patient education • Preop care • Postop care • Day of surgery

KEY POINTS

- Patients seeking surgery for rejuvenation for the first time are initially uninformed.
- Patient education is critical in achieving excellent outcomes.
- The surgery is just one part of successful outcomes.
- Care begins with the first phone call to schedule an appointment.
- Care ends with the last postop appointment 1 year later.

A PERSONAL APPROACH CULTIVATED OVER 45 YEARS OF DOING REJUVENATION SURGERY

It is important for the facial plastic surgeon to focus beyond the technical aspects of rejuvenation surgery to have a very successful outcome. The entire experience from the first "Hello" to the last "Goodbye" must be carefully crafted to achieve as near a perfect outcome as possible. Patients have a general sense of the work of a facial plastic surgeon by speaking with friends who have had work done by the doctor, from reviews, social media, and online research. Issues that are of considerable importance to most patients include possible risks, likely sequelae, bandages, drains, bruising, pain, and when normal activities can be resumed. Rapid and uneventful recovery along with excellent results will be one of the practice's best marketing tools.[1]

Surgery is the "great unknown" for most people. The word is fraught with mystery. Generally, surgery is done out of exigent or emergent necessity. The idea of being unconscious from anesthesia and being "cut open" can be at the very least disconcerting and at the worst frightening. Most cannot fathom having a desire to be operated on. For the most part, the cohort of patients desiring facial rejuvenation is aware that surgery may be recommended for their desires to be fulfilled. That written, today there is a plethora of noninvasive and minimally invasive options available that are often sufficient enough to meet the expectations of many patients. When surgery is the desired and indicated option, there is still a cloud of uncertainty and anxiety that occupies space in the patient's psyche that ebbs and flows until the date of the procedure.

There are 2 important and intertwined factors that result in successful outcomes. One is the skill and technical talent of the facial plastic surgeon and the other is the perceived outcome in the eyes of the patient having undergone rejuvenative surgery as well as in the eyes of the surgeon.

[a] Division of Otolaryngology–Head and Neck Surgery, University of Connecticut School of Medicine, Farmington, CT, USA; [b] American Board of Facial Plastic and Reconstructive Surgery; [c] American Academy of Facial Plastic and Reconstructive Surgery; [d] Private Practice, Easthampton, MA, USA
* 123 Union Street, Suite 100, Easthampton, MA 01027.
E-mail address: bill.truswell@gmail.com

Facial Plast Surg Clin N Am 28 (2020) 429–436
https://doi.org/10.1016/j.fsc.2020.06.001
1064-7406/20/© 2020 Elsevier Inc. All rights reserved.

> **Box 1**
> **Typical desires and worries of facial plastic surgery patients**
>
> - Can I trust this surgeon?
> - Will this surgeon listen to my concerns?
> - How good is this surgeon's work?
> - How much experience does this surgeon have?
> - What if something horrible happens?
> - What if I don't like the result?
> - Will 1 still look like me?
> - Will people notice? Will people stare?
> - How long will it last?
> - How much will it cost?

Hessler and colleagues published an early study examining factors that may predict patient satisfaction with cosmetic surgery results. Patients who are more likely to be pleased with their outcomes include men, older patients, patients with higher education experiences, and those who have not had previous cosmetic surgery.[2]

THE BEGINNING

The goal of every operation should be, "Were the patient's desires met and was the surgeon proud of the result?". The perception of many patients is that surgery itself is gruesome involving cutting, lifting, and removing, a procedure fraught with blood, pain, and bandages. For them, the road from start to finish can be unpleasant and frightening. **Box 1** is a list of some concerns new patients have at the start (see **Box 1**). The responsibility of the facial plastic surgeon is to make their experience as safe, pleasant, and tranquil as possible. The patient is generally well aware of her appearance and what she would like to have improved. **Fig. 1** is a graphic representation of the of the ideal mental process that we would like the patient to have (see **Fig. 1**). She knows what she sees in the mirror and what she would like the outcome to be after all is said and done. Ideally, on that road from consultation to the postoperative photographs, the patient will develop an understanding of the ease of the journey and not be consumed by images of incisions, stitches, swelling, pain, disfigurement, and complications.

The infrastructure of any successful practice is the office staff. Each staff member must be a people friendly person. They must enjoy interpersonal interaction and should have warm, inviting, and cheerful personalities. From start to finish, patient education is the cornerstone of successful and happy outcomes. Patient education starts with the first phone call to the surgeon's office. The call must be answered promptly by a friendly, cheerful, and pleasant person who is inviting and informative and takes time to answer questions to the best of his/her abilities. The receptionist must have a special skill set. She/he needs to be a "people person." She/he must enjoy engaging with a stranger, have the innate ability to make the patient feel welcome, and feel as if her call were important to the practice. The entire office staff should become the patients' cosmetic surgery "family." They need to embrace each patient and foster a sense of carrying and deep concern for each one. The patients need to feel they can call or even drop in and that they will be warmly greeted by every staff member they may encounter. They will not be rushed but listened to and their questions will be answered honestly and freely.

On the day of the first consultation, the patient should be greeted by a friendly staffer and welcomed to the office. The setting should be comfortable, inviting, and nonclinical (**Fig. 2**). Paperwork will need to be filled out and it should be as brief as possible, and the patient should not have to sit for a long wait for the next step. All physicians have their personal styles that work successfully for them. As an example, in my office, when these preliminaries are finished, the patient is greeted by Lynn, my office manager, lawyer, and wife, who starts the conversation by getting to know the patient with friendly conversation. She employs questions about where the patient lives, comments about the ever changing New England seasons, or how the Red Sox/Patriots are doing. The approach is designed to put her at ease by chatting about everyday items. The goals are to never rush the encounter, foster a friendly and familiar atmosphere, and start building a relationship based on trust. Their conversation is gently eased into the concerns the patient has about her appearance. Having had 25 years, first as a psychologist and then attorney, Lynn is very insightful in reading a person's character and evaluating her as a prospective surgical candidate. This is done in a small office that is intimate, nicely appointed, and nonclinical. When the rapport is established, Lynn takes the patient's photographs.

Lynn asks the patient to wait a moment to see if I am ready. She and I then have a brief conversation. Lynn tells me of her assessment of the patient's goals, whether the patient seems to have

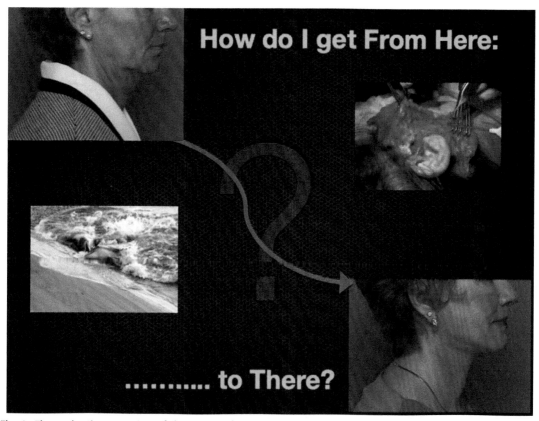

Fig. 1. The patient's perception of the journey from start to finish.

roalictic expectation, and understands the services we offer. I also have a quick look at the medical history provided on our intake sheet.

Then she escorts the patient to my consultation office and introduces us. My office reflects my personal taste and is comfortable and inviting (**Fig. 3**). The patient sits on a small couch and I in a chair positioned diagonally across and relatively close

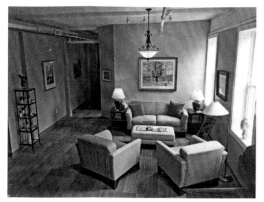

Fig. 2. The waiting room is warm, comfortable, and nonclinical.

to her. At the consultation, I also chat with her asking where she lives, what she does, and so on. It is a friendly conversation as one would have in a social setting. It is all designed to maintain and nurture the personal relationship that was fostered when she entered our front door. I want her to get a sense of me, my character, and personality. At the end of our consultation I want to answer this question for the patient, "Can I trust this doctor?", and I want to answer this question for me, "Is this patient a suitable candidate for surgery?" (**Fig. 4**).

After this informal talk, I start the consultation by asking "What concerns would you like me to address?". In one form or another, some may voice that they only are interested in nonsurgical treatments. Others may state that I am the expert and what would I advise. I take my cue from the comments and from watching their body language. Often, while they are answering, their hands wander to their cheeks and push upward in spite of averring, for example, that they are only interested in their eyelids. It seems clear that the lower face is an issue. I then have her stand facing a window. I examine her with daylight using a mirror as I feel warranted. I believe it is important

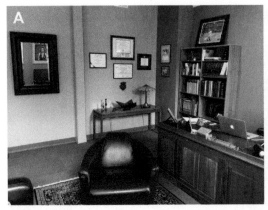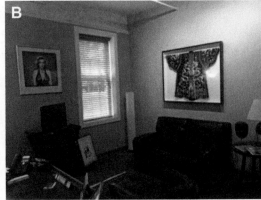

Fig. 3. (*A, B*) Consultation office. Pleasant and reflecting my personal tastes and interests.

to touch her face, gently lifting her cheeks and brow. I believe touch is important. It communicates the confidence I have in my hands. And touch is symbolic of healing which we, as doctors, do after all.

Returning to our seats, I discuss how the female face ages. I discuss the skin, sagging of tissues, and volume loss. I mention that a woman's face becomes more masculine over time in that men have coarse skin, low brows, thin lips, square jawlines, and heavy necks. Living in a less ostentatious part of the country where folks do not necessarily want to draw attention to themselves, I add that I feel my job is to refresh, rejuvenate, and refeminize the face and that it should be age appropriate. I have found that this conversation has been very successful in my practice over very many years. **Box 2** lists a

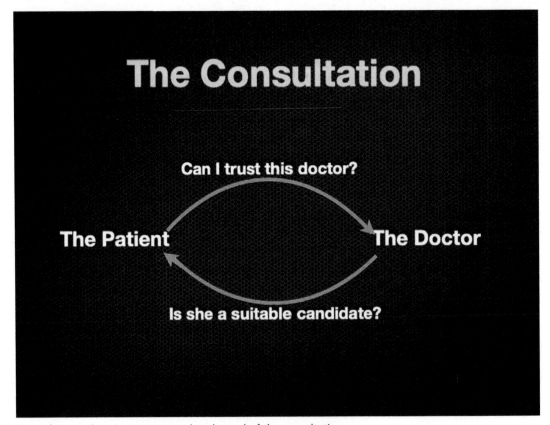

Fig. 4. The questions I want answered at the end of the consultation.

few pearls that help me connect with the patient (see **Box 2**).

The next step is for us to look at her photographs. If she has stated that she is only interested in her eyes or nonsurgical procedures, I ask her if she would like me to discuss all that I see. Most patients do. I show her the lateral photograph first and say, "Let's change the picture some." I perform computer imaging as I describe what can be done. Then I take her through albums of my patients addressing her specific concerns. I show photographs from 1 week postop to a decade later and patients from their 40s to their 80s, men as well as women. I make a point of showing the incisions on many of the patients. During this discussion, I address that the surgery is done in office in my operating suite, which is accredited by American Association for Accreditation of Ambulatory Surgery Facilities, and explain what that means. I discuss the conscious sedation administered by Certified Registered Nurse Anesthetists (CRNAs). I describe the dressing and the fact that I do not use drains. It is important to discuss that although there may be some discomfort and stiffness, there is little to no significant pain. They understand the dressing is removed the next day and their hair will be washed, a sling will be supplied, and that all sutures will dissolve on their own in 6 or 7 days. They understand the cheeks will be numb, feel stiff to touch, and the ear will be numb as well for a period of weeks or longer. All possible complications and sequalae are outlined in detail as gently as possible. Smokers are informed in particular about the inherent negative effects of tobacco use on the healing process. They are strongly advised to cease at least 2 weeks before the surgery date,

and the risk of smoking to the healing process is discussed in detail. Another issue I explore is a history of keloid or hypertrophic scar formation. If that is positive, I inform the patient that it could be problematic and afterward if it seems to be occurring there are means to deal with it. I do have them understand that they are accepting some of the responsibility for such a happenstance if we proceed. After all her questions are answered and she wishes to schedule a procedure, Lynn will meet with her again to discuss the financial issues and book a convenient date for her. It is not uncommon that Lynn will get more questions from the patient at that juncture, and either I or the nurse will address them before she leaves.

THREE WEEKS BEFORE SURGERY

This is the formal preoperative appointment with a nurse. This is the next major step in patient education. She will spend up to an hour, as needed, with the patient. The entire process is designed to educate the patient and make her confident about her decision to become a partner with us on this journey to rejuvenation. It is important that the patient understands she has certain duties and obligations that will contribute to a successful outcome and happy result.

If the surgery has been scheduled months ahead, I will do a reconsult as well. All our clinical discussions are preceded by informal and personal chats reestablishing the "family" relationship. The nurse discusses all the perioperative and postoperative procedures with the patient and the basic instructions such as don't bend over, don't lift anything heavier than a box of tissues, do not do housekeeping chores, such as vacuuming, loading the dishwasher, cooking, laundry, etc. The patient is shown the sling she will wear the week following removal of her dressing. The importance of the use of cold compresses is discussed. Smokers are strongly advised to cease at least 2 weeks before the surgery date, and the risks of smoking to the healing process are reviewed again. Written prescriptions are given and reviewed. We use an antibiotic, an analgesic with the strong suggestion that all that is really needed is acetaminophen, an antiviral and antifungal if concomitant CO_2 fractional laser resurfacing will be done, and a sleeping aid if desired for the night before and morning of surgery. The nurse also reviews how and when the patient can shower, how to do simple wound care, and what clothing to wear the morning of surgery. The time to arrive for the procedure is set. The anesthesia, conscious sedation, is described. A list of over-the-counter pills and supplements

---

Box 2
Some rules for the consultation

- Be humble, show no conceit
- Establish rapport
- Assess her needs, personality, self-awareness, character
- "What brought you here?"—observe her hands
- Examine with minor—ask and use gentle touch
- Examine with imaging—do not show more than you can deliver
- Share examples of the work you do
- Discuss the risks, both sequelae and complications

and certain foods that can promote bleeding are reviewed.

All of this information is printed and placed into the patient's preop folder that she will take with her. If the patient routinely has her hair colored, we recommend it be done no sooner than 1 week before the day of surgery, and we strongly urge the patient not to do so until 1 month after the procedure. Patients who live more than an hour's drive distant are required to stay locally the night of the procedure. There is an inn near us that accommodates our patients and offers a discounted rate. We make those arrangements for the patients. We also require that the patient must have a friend or family member stay with them the night of surgery. When that is not possible, we arrange for a health care worker to be hired.

THE OPERATIVE AND PERIOPERATIVE DAYS

The day before surgery, the nurse calls the patient to put her at ease, inform her that we will take very good care of her and that she is important to us. They review the pre- and postoperative instructions again, what type of clothing to wear, when to arrive, and what will happen the next day.

When they arrive the next morning, the nurse is there to greet the patient warmly, meet her care giver, offer reassuring words to the companion, get his/her phone number, and tell him/her approximately what time to return or when the surgeon will call. The patient is taken to the presurgery room and changes into a surgical gown. The nurse reviews the procedure and goals, tells the patient that the doctor will mark her face in another room, and that anesthesia will interview her afterward. There is no rushing, no confusion, all is calm. I see her in an examination room next and chat for a few minutes, review, once again, the procedure and its goals, that the bandage will be in place when she awakes, and that there will be little discomfort. With the patient sitting, I mark her face and continue the conversation. Back in the preop area, she is greeted by anesthesia who reviews the surgery, her medical history, and does a brief physical examination.

Anesthetist walks the patient into the operating room (OR) and introduces her to the nurses who pause their chores to welcome and reassure her that we will take good care of her. We keep the OR at a comfortable temperature until the patient is sedated. We use a warming blanket and, after she is quiet, lower the room temperature to our comfort level. Likewise, we increase the temperature as the patient is coming to. What happens in the OR is crucial to the patient's perception and outcome. With local anesthesia, conscious, and likely general anesthesia, the patient will input sounds, noises, and even conversation. It is important to use nonalarming speech. Words that are part of our daily lives can frighten a patient in the surgical setting. Avoiding terms such as "knife, scalpel, cut here, a bleeder," etc., if at all possible. Try to avoid speaking in loud, rushed, urgent, or worried fashion. What is normal for us can produce unintended psychological consequences in the patient. With conscious sedation the patient may "lighten up" and, unbeknownst to us, hear what is being said.[3] If you are talking about the Super Bowl, she might wonder why you are not paying attention to her. And if you say "sponge, quick, etc." she might misinterpret that something is going wrong.

We play quiet music in surgery and ask the patient what type, if any, she prefers. We keep the atmosphere calm and quiet with the alarms minimized and the activity unrushed. The circulating nurse holds the patient's hand and quietly talks with her while the intravenous is started IV and conscious sedation is started. The nurses apply the dressing quickly and gently as the patient wakes up. With conscious sedation, generally a combination of propofol and versed, patients awaken quickly and smoothly and experience a sense of wellbeing. When ready, the CRNA and circulator walk the patient to the postanesthesia

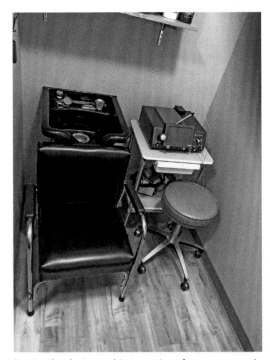

Fig. 5. The hair washing station for postoperative patients.

care unit. They are partially reclined in a Geri chair. Soft music is playing. The companion sits with her until she is settled in and comfortable. And when ready she receives something light to eat and drink. The nurses look in on her at 10-minute intervals. Most patients are ready to leave within an hour. Before discharge, the nurse reviews the written instructions with the care giver who receives a second copy. The evening of the procedure the nurse calls the patient to check on her status and reassure all went well, and we will see her in the morning.

The following day, the patient arrives and comes in a side door so that she can avoid the waiting room and any curious glances. My nurse gently removes the dressing and cleans the incisions. She then washes and blow dries the patient's hair. We use a hair washing station installed in a clinical room (**Fig. 5**). I have found that to be a big bonus for patients. They are concerned about their hair. It feels good to have it washed and is a "normal" activity after all that happened over the preceding 24 hours. The patient then sees how she looks in a 3-way mirror. My nurse again stresses the most important postoperative instructions—no straining, head

elevated, avoid blood thinners, etc. I come in to see my patient after all is done and examine her, tell her she looks terrific only 24 hours after surgery, and briefly reaffirm she understands her duties going forward. Her companion is brought in and instructed in how to care for the incisions. An elastic-like sling is applied and ice bags are provided. It is emphasized that "ice is your friend" especially for the first 3 days and for as long as it feels good. The sling is to be worn continuously for 3 days and then it can be removed for meals and to take showers. After 3 days, she can gently wash her hair in the shower with tepid water and a mild shampoo. The nurse sees the patient on the fourth or fifth day postop. She returns on day 8 to see me and my nurse to answer questions and perform any needed wound care. The sling will be used at nighttime for an additional week. After 2 weeks, she can begin to resume normal activities except vigorous exercise. After 3 weeks mild exercise can commence gradually, increasing the intensity over the ensuing week. She returns at 6 weeks for a "makeover" with the aesthetician who also councils on a skin care program going forward. Further visits are scheduled at 3,6, and 12 months or as needed.

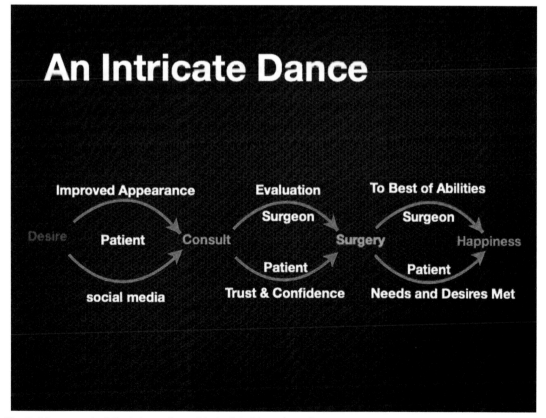

Fig. 6. My concept of that dance from "desire" to" happiness."

Patients living at a distance will have a convenient return schedule as practical.

SUMMARY

I believe it is important to keep in mind that in our profession, we meet a stranger, spend half an hour or more talking with her, and work to convince her that there is no reason for us to not take knife and scissor and cut her face to change the way she looks. That establishes trust and that trust will enable us to build a relationship with our patients that will enable us to help them feel better about themselves—that's no small thing. Remember, "I trust you" can almost be a better compliment than "I love you" because you may not always trust the person you love, but you can always love the person you trust." It is also important to understand that our patients are not ill, do not need surgery for their physical wellbeing, and are willing to undergo completely elective surgery to improve their appearance. They want and need to trust us. It is up to us to create our own method to engender that feeling.

Every surgeon has his/her own approach to guiding his/her patients on this wonderful journey of facial rejuvenation. I see this interaction as a well-choreographed dance between surgeon, patient, and staff (**Fig. 6**). The surgeon may lead the dance, but the dance ends when the patient has an excellent outcome and feels as if her rejuvenated face enhances her powerful personal perception! There is no perfect nor universal formula in how to do it. We accomplish our own formulas for this by learning from our mentors, networking with colleagues, and reading journals. Eventually the maturing facial plastic surgeon grows into the dance that best suits his/her practice. **Fig. 5** illustrates my concept of that dance from "desire" to "happiness" (see **Fig. 6**).

DISCLOSURE

The author has nothing to disclose.

REFERENCES

1. Zimbler MS, Mashkevic G. Pearls in facelift management. Facial Plast Surg Clin North Am 2009;17(4): 625–32.
2. Hessler JL, Moyer CA, Kim JC, et al. Predictors of satisfaction with facial plastic surgery: results of a prospective study. Arch Facial Plast Surg 2010; 12(3):192–6.
3. Hom DB. Enhancing the art of care during awake procedures. Arch Facial Plast Surg 2014;7(1):5–6.

Incorporating Nonsurgical Options and Aesthetic Services into Your Facial Plastic Surgery Practice

Catherine Winslow, MD

KEYWORDS

• Nonsurgical • Skin care • Chemical peels • Aesthetician

KEY POINTS

- Nonsurgical services can improve patient satisfaction, longevity of surgical procedures, and office revenue stream.
- Many options exist for both physician and ancillary staff to provide skin-care and nonsurgical treatments and product.
- An optimal approach to offering nonsurgical services can involve low overhead, a good profit margin, and simple startup options.

The ability of facial plastic surgeons to improve patient satisfaction and outcomes is greatly amplified by incorporating nonsurgical services and product into a practice. Such additions can be immensely gratifying, both personally and financially, but should be approached with a broad understanding of what is entailed in such a venture to avoid costly mistakes. Bringing in new products and services can be fun, exciting, and rewarding when approached correctly. Although some schools of thought and even previous American Medical Association admonitions have looked at product sales and been wary of encroaching on the patient-physician relationship,[1] there is no one better able to provide expert information and recommendations than a provider school in skin physiology.

The US skin-care market is projected to reach around \$11 billion in 2018[2] and continues to grow, with a small percentage of clients and over-the-counter brands comprising the overwhelming majority of sales. Physicians offering skin-care products as well as services, to include sunscreens, moisturizers, potent serums, and cleansers, can not only improve global patient care but also improve revenue streams.[3] Skin-care procedures can nicely complement surgical antiaging procedures by enhancing collagen, elastic, and minimizing dark spots and fine lines. Nonsurgical procedures can be performed by skin-care specialists (aestheticians), nurses, or physicians, although state laws vary with regards to regulating certain procedures by license (for example, neurotoxins may be injected only by a doctor or nurse in some states but may not be regulated in others). It is important before adding nonsurgical options to a practice to fully explore legal implications and state and federal laws that regulate such practices.

Nonsurgical options are varied and almost endless. Those most commonly chosen are selected to improve skin appearance mildly with products and aesthetic services, more dramatically improve the skin with physician-administered skin services, or delay or augment surgical procedures with neurotoxins and injectable fillers.

IU School of Medicine, Winslow Facial Plastic Surgery, 2000 East 116th Street, Suite 200, Carmel, IN 46032, USA
E-mail address: drwinslow@indyface.com

Facial Plast Surg Clin N Am 28 (2020) 437–442
https://doi.org/10.1016/j.fsc.2020.06.002

AESTHETIC SERVICES

Nonsurgical skin-care options can be enhanced by adding a skin-care professional, such as an aesthetician, to a practice. An aesthetician is a licensed professional who goes through training to be able to identify and treat facial cosmetic concerns with epidermal treatments and product. The opportunity to build clients to improve and maintain skin health as well as make personal recommendations regarding skin type–specific products can improve the ability to offer comprehensive antiaging services and enhance patient satisfaction. Nonsurgical options are varied, and some may require additional training for personnel, including the typical procedures listed in **Table 1**.

Startup considerations include equipment, space, and personnel. The initial investment is usually minimal to moderate, but it may take time to develop an active practice and note continued return on initial investment. One room with a bed that reclines, a sink, back-bar product, supplies, and storage is required for each aesthetician. Additional equipment, such as a micro-dermabrasion machine, can be added quickly. Hiring the right aesthetician is the key to success, and finding a well-trained individual who blends well with the office staff is crucial. The pay for aestheticians varies greatly depending on region and experience. Options of hourly pay, commission, or combined bring different benefits for the aesthetician and physician. Salary is attractive for a starting aesthetician who may need a guaranteed financial base until an active clientele is established. More seasoned aestheticians who bring their own client base benefit more from straight commission, or a pay schedule that is heavier on commission than salary. Most offices will start at no more than 40% to 50% commission if provided commission only for pay, with the commission going down as hourly pay increases. It is crucial to ensure the pay structure allows for profit on the end of the physician, even when accounting for disposables, product, overhead, and equipment. It is equally important to analyze patient retention and aesthetician profitability on a regular basis.

Treatment options offered by an aesthetician will vary based on skill and state laws regulating the scope of aesthetic practices. Most states limit the role of the aesthetician to the epidermis, and procedures that penetrate into the subdermal tissues would be out of the scope of their license. Aestheticians are taught to perform facials, light peels, and micro-dermabrasion in their training. Additional services, such as dermaplaning, light-based therapies, and microneedling, require additional instruction and certification. Solutions for light peels, including Jessner's, glycolic acid, lactic acid, and other fruit-based acids, are easily obtained by most medical-grade skin-care companies and companies that specialize in peel mixtures (such as Delasco, Council Bluffs, IA, USA). Results of aesthetic treatments are subtle and are designed to help with skin maintenance more than significant rejuvenation. These treatments, as with surgical

Table 1
Common aesthetic services

Procedure	Description
Dermaplaning	A blade edge removes facial vellus hairs and dead skin cells, resulting in exfoliation and a smooth skin surface
Micro-dermabrasion	A crystal or diamond tip applicator abrades and removes epithelial cells
Superficial chemical peels	Fruit acid peels, such as lactic acids, as well as Jessner's solution or low concentrations of TCA allow chemical burn and removal of epithelial cells, hyperpigmentation, and fine lines
Facial	A relaxing treatment intended to soothe and hydrate the skin, often combined with other procedures, such as light peels or dermaplaning
Microneedling	A rolling device with fine needles penetrates the outer dermis to enhance collagen and elastin deposition
Waxing	Hot wax allows for precise removal of facial hair
Additional services	Procedures, such as lash tinting or lifting, brow tinting, lash extensions, and other cosmetic procedures, add to satisfaction
Intense pulsed light/lasers	Improve dark spots and fine lines and resurface or tighten skin
Microblading	Semipermanent pigment deposition typically used for brow darkening

procedures, are improved with the addition of a skin-care regimen with quality products.

Skin-care products can be added with or without an aesthetician, although it helps office flow to have staff that is knowledgeable about skin questions and products. Having the staff use the marketed product lines for sale is a valuable tool to promote internal marketing. Product options are diverse and often marketed directly to physicians. Both prescription and nonprescription strength products can improve the ability to maintain the outcomes of surgical procedures. Initial investment in products can be costly, and an assessment of patient load and purchasing predictions (business plan) are helpful, especially if financing will be required for startup. There are many product lines from which to choose, and most offer a vast array of treatment options for different skin conditions. As the nonsurgical practice grows, the skin-care line may also need to expand. When planning options for skin-care products, it is important to consider not just ingredients but also application. Most commonly, a skin-care routine will include a cleanser, moisturizer, sunscreen, and possibly a serum or toner. Products are typically designed either for a skin type: dry, oily, or combination, or for a problem, such as aging, pigment, or acne. Prescription skin-care products, such as tretinoin (vitamin A) or hydroquinone, may fall under state regulations, which should be explored before offering these to patients. The use of hydroquinone has significantly decreased in the past decade and is banned in several countries because of the potential carcinogenic effects. Other bleaching agents, such as kojic acid, arbutin, and vitamin C, have been promoted as front-line agents for skin lightening and treatment of hyperpigmentation. Many product lines offer incentives linked to injectables or other company purchases, but these also may be more widely available in the area. Products should be displayed in a secured but aesthetic fashion in a heavily trafficked area for maximum in-house marketing benefit. Sampling is effective in encouraging patients to "feel" and experience the product while having an opportunity to ask questions. Patients should always have recommendations of product and services printed out for future reference.

One of the most important skin-care products that can be offered is sunscreen. It is important to educate patients on the value and differences in sunscreen, what sun protection factor (SPF) means, and what sunscreen will and will not do. Sunscreens will not block all UV light and will not cause vitamin D deficiency, even when correctly applied and frequently reapplied.[4] Zinc oxide and titanium dioxide are common components that are both reef-safe (important in vacation planning) and give a physical block of UV A and B rays, thus protecting against accelerated aging as well as skin cancer. Nanoparticles are commonly used to make the sunscreen clear and less pasty, but such small particles have been noted to interrupt growth of hair follicles and are optimally avoided. Sunscreens with an SPF higher than 50 typically offer no additional benefit, but reapplication of sunscreen no matter the SPF is crucial to minimize risk of burns and skin cancer. Sunscreens are available in tinted and nontinted formulations, powders, creams, and sprays, making options available for every skin type and preference.

Every skin-care plan should include an antioxidant and a moisturizer. Some form of exfoliation is very helpful but should always be accompanied by replenishing the moisture of the skin surface to minimize irritation, and exfoliation should never be overdone. A simple fruit acid, vitamin A derivative, or treatment such as dermaplaning will take care of exfoliation needs. Antioxidants can be added based on skin type and program. The most common and effective antioxidants include vitamin C, vitamin E, green tea, and resveratrol. Most skin-care lines will carry a variety of options, from serums to creams, that include one or several antioxidants. Vitamin A derivatives can be over the counter or more effective prescription strength but should not be used in patients who are pregnant, trying to get pregnant, or breast feeding.

NONSURGICAL MEDICAL SERVICES

Nonsurgical services can be offered as a "liquid facelift" and are largely lumped together as neuromodulators, injectable fillers, and skin resurfacing options (**Table 2**). Injectables can often be administered by nurses or physician extenders (nurse practitioners or physician assistants) depending on state laws. Skin resurfacing that is ablative, to include 35% trichloracetic acid (TCA) peels, is most commonly considered under the domain of the surgeon. Neuromodulators remain the most common nonsurgical procedure in both men and women[5] followed by injectable fillers to restore volume. Several injectable filler options exist in the United States, but the most commonly used are the hyaluronic acid family. Both neurotoxins and injectable fillers are temporary. One must be cautious labeling any injectable filler as "permanent" because it can mislead the patient to think no further fillers will ever be needed, neglecting the physiology of continued aging.

Neuromodulators are injected with a small needle into muscles of facial expression, most commonly in the periorbital region. Temporary complications,

Table 2
Additional nonsurgical options

Outcome	Options
Volumize	Fillers
Minimize dynamic rhytids	Neuromodulators
Remove fat	Injectable deoxycholic acid, fat freezing devices
Skin tightening	Medium to deep chemical peels, light-based devices/lasers, ultrasound devices, microneedling/microneedling with radiofrequency
Treat hyperpigmentation	Medium to deep chemical peels, lasers
Ablative resurfacing	Medium to deep chemical peels, Er-Yag or CO_2 laser, dermabrasion

such as eyelid ptosis, are rare and reflect an injection too deep and proximal to the levator muscle. Bruising is uncommon, but avoidance of anti-inflammatory medications and supplements can minimize the risk. Results take 5 to 10 days and last approximately 3 months. The physician's initial purchase of a vial of neuromodulator is not inexpensive, but patient demand is high, and the potential for a moderate return on investment is good for most areas. Although neuromodulators may be reimbursable in the treatment of headaches or hyperhidrosis, most treatments are cosmetic. Insurance reimbursements may not cover the cost of the neurotoxin vial, and many physicians are wary of billing for these procedures because of the high initial vial cost. Neuromodulators have recently been noted to be associated with an improvement in elasticity and viscoelastic properties in the skin on a histologic level.[6] This added benefit may improve the youthful dermal maintenance and promote skin longevity. They have also been used to improve surgical results, often injected several weeks before surgery to help set brow position and improve symmetry of results[7] or minimize fine lines and pull against the healing incisions postoperatively.

Injectable fillers are injected for volumetric enhancement, most commonly in the perioral area and lower face. Filler placement requires more training than neurotoxins for excellent results, and often different types of fillers can be layered for optimal outcomes. Injectable fillers are often preceded by topical numbing, and like neuromodulators, can cause bruising. They also have a risk of vascular occlusion and skin necrosis, a rare but devastating occurrence treated with immediate hyaluronidase flooding, warm compresses, and massage. Technique and experience are crucial to optimal results.

Nonsurgical options can be expanded with additional expense to options that improve skin tone, volume, color, and elasticity. Options range from inexpensive peels to light-based therapies requiring more significant investments. Return on investment is crucial to consider before making any large purchase, and a business plan is a valuable asset in planning. Speaking with physicians who own similar systems, trialing any equipment, and ensuring adequate staffing and space are imperative before making a purchase.

Light-based therapies and options are extensive and covered well in other publications. Such platforms offer results that often can be achieved at a fraction of the startup cost of other modalities. Other less expensive options for resurfacing, including medium and deep peels and dermabrasion, have largely fallen by the wayside despite decades of research, success, and patient satisfaction. These techniques offer the surgeon a virtual 100% profit margin and require minimal training. Dermabrasion requires minimal investment with a dermabrader machine and wands, although some surgeons have reported using sterile sandpaper with equivalent results.[8] Deep peels typically involve phenol, which can be toxic to the heart, liver, and kidneys and requires sedation. Medium-depth peels, such as Jessner's 35% TCA, can be performed without sedation at no risk to organs and with predictable, safe results. Medium-depth peels improve skin elasticity, fine lines, and hyperpigmentation in a more dramatic fashion than aesthetic treatments and with very minimal investment and learning curve required. Medium-depth peels have also been shown to reduce skin tumor formation associated with UV light exposure.[9]

ACHIEVING SUCCESS WITH NONSURGICAL SERVICES

Although nonsurgical options are commonly found in most facial plastics practices, the variety from which to choose is almost endless. Achieving success with the addition to the practice requires a definition of goals as well as a thorough strategic plan for marketing.

Goals of adding practice components may include financial gain, improving patient flow, improving patient satisfaction, or all of the above. If financial gain is the primary objective, then options with low startup costs and overhead that are easy to market and not widely available should be targeted. Patient volume is optimized by adding options with high levels of name recognition or current use but may require more marketing to distinguish the practice from a widely available service. Improving patient satisfaction may require a focus on services that will complete but not compete with surgical services currently offered, with aesthetic follow-up and treatments a critical component.

With any new venture, legalities of the proposed plan should first be evaluated by competent counsel for assurance that all state and federal regulations are being followed. Many skin-care product manufacturers have restrictions regarding discount levels and online marketing, which should be understood before committing to a skin-care line. State laws often dictate what level of provider is required for specific equipment.

Marketing is essential to the success of any venture. Both internal and external marketing should be used and taught to all employees. Internal marketing takes advantage of an aesthetic client base and can incorporate print ads prominently displayed, video graphics, photo books, samples, and brochures. External marketing is turning more and more to social media options, such as Instagram and Facebook. Posts by employees and patients alike can boost visibility and provide powerful and inexpensive marketing advantages.

From the time the patient walks through the door, they will form an impression of the experience that can help you assess any small details previously not considered. An easy way to prevent this is to perform a mock-up of the experience, using the provider and a "sample" patient, preferably one who is friendly to the practice, or a staff member who can understand the impressions given. Consideration should be given from start (lobby appearance, check-in process and paperwork, and reception staff) to the actual service provided. Planning from a 360° viewpoint can identify issues not previously considered and optimize flow and success. Products should have a prominent yet secure position in the office and have good lighting (**Fig. 1**). Brochures of services should feature faces that are attractive and representative of the client base. A pleasant reception staff and office environment are crucial to success. Patient retention is the goal, and follow-up calls or visits assist in promoting continued loyalty to the office.

SUMMARY

The addition of nonsurgical services to an existing practice, or addition of 1 arm of these services, can increase practice profitability while improving patient satisfaction and treatment goals. A thoughtful approach to such additions is required in order to avoid speed bumps that can lead to loss of patients and profit. Old-school concepts of interference with patient-physician relationship through product sales have largely been supplanted by the concept of the physician's office as a business. With the knowledge, experience, and options available to facial plastics surgeons, there is no one better suited to provide medical-grade skin-care options and a full range of nonsurgical services to augment what surgical skills can accomplish and maintain optimal results.

REFERENCES

1. Slade K, Grant-Kels JM. Employing an aesthetician in a dermatology practice: facts and controversies. Clin Dermatol 2013;31(6):777–9.
2. Available at: Blog.marketresearch.com.
3. Austin RE, Ahmad J, Lista F. The impact of skin care product sales in an aesthetic plastic surgery practice. Aesthet Surg J 2020;40(3):330–4.

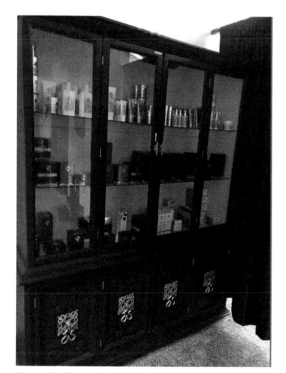

Fig. 1. Products should have a prominent yet secure position in the office and have good lighting.

4. Passeron T, Bouillon R, Callender V, et al. Sunscreen photoprotection and vitamin D status. Br J Deramtol 2019;181(5):916–31.

5. Available at: https://www.aafprs.org/media/stats_polls/m_stats.html.

6. Bonaparte JP, Ellis D. Alterations in the elasticity, pliability and viscoelastic properties of facial skin after injection of onabotulinum toxin A. JAMA Facial Plast Surg 2015;17(4):256–63.

7. Sweis IE, Hwang L, Cohen M. Preoperative use of neuromodulators to optimize surgical outcomes in upper blepharoplasty and brow lift. Aesthet Surg J 2018;38(9):941–8.

8. Pavlidis L, Spyropoulou GA. A simple technique to perform manual dermabrasion with sandpaper. Dermatol Surg 2012;38(12):2016–7.

9. Abdel-Daim M, Funasaka Y, Kamo T, et al. Preventive effect of chemical peeling on ultraviolet induced skin tumor formation. J Dermatol Sci 2010;60(1):21–8.

Evaluating, Purchasing, and Incorporating High-Tech Equipment into a Facial Plastic Surgery Practice

Richard D. Gentile, MD, MBA[a,b,*]

KEYWORDS

- Skin rejuvenation • Facial contouring • Skin tightening • Facial tissue • Energy-based devices
- Electrosurgical • Plasma technology

KEY POINTS

- Energy has been applied in some form to tissue since the beginning of recorded history. The practice of applying heat to tissue with the use of cauters was used for thousands of years as an invaluable method of controlling hemorrhage.
- In October 1926, Dr Harvey Cushing used an electrosurgical unit developed by Dr William T. Bovie to successfully remove a highly vascularized brain tumor from a patient after previous failed attempts.
- The end of collagen contraction and skin tightening occurs in the last phase of wound healing, as realignment of collagen bundles permits overall contraction of the soft tissue and skin mass to occur.
- The types of procedures possible have significantly increased over the past 20 years since the advent of skin tightening devices, and technology-assisted procedures are the fastest growing segment of facial rejuvenation procedures.

METHODS OF ENERGY-BASED SKIN REJUVENATION

The market for nonsurgical, energy-based facial rejuvenation techniques has increased exponentially since lasers were first used for skin rejuvenation in 1983, and the concept of selective photothermolysis was presented.[1,2] Advances in this area have led to a wide range of devices that require the modern skin rejuvenation specialists to have a large repertoire of knowledge. Three broad categories of technology are leading nonenergy-based rejuvenation technology: lasers, light therapy, and nonlaser-based thermal tightening devices. Laser light therapy has continued to diversify with the use of ablative and nonablative resurfacing technologies, fractionated lasers, and their combined use. Broad band light therapy has been developed for use in combination with other technologies or stand alone. Finally, thermally based nonlaser skin-tightening devices, such as radiofrequency (RF) and intense focused ultrasonography, are evolving technologies that have changed rapidly over the past 5 years. Plasma technologies are new entries to the current assortment of devices and were initially introduced at the beginning of this millennium nearly 20 years ago. These devices use different medium for plasma generation including some using saline, but most plasma systems use noble gases for the purposes of ionization and plasma generation. Nitrogen plasma was first introduced about 15 years ago[2,3] and Renuvion (RF-HeP) (**Fig. 1**) is the most recent plasma device introduced and

[a] Facial Plastic Surgery, Gentile Facial Plastic Surgery & Aesthetic Laser Center, 821 Kentwood Suite C, Youngstown, OH 44512, USA; [b] Facial Plastic Surgery, Cleveland Clinic Akron General Hospital, Akron, OH, USA
* 821 Kentwood Suite C, Youngstown, OH 44512.
E-mail address: dr-gentile@msn.com

Facial Plast Surg Clin N Am 28 (2020) 443–450
https://doi.org/10.1016/j.fsc.2020.07.005

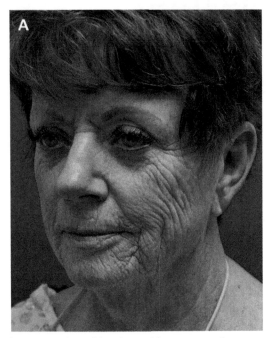 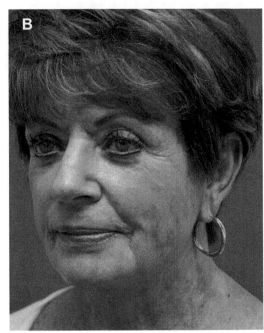

Fig. 1. A 75-year-old patient with severe sun damage and rhytides treated with RF-HeP (Renuvion) shown before (*A*) and 4 months after procedure (*B*).

approved by Food and Drug Administration (FDA) in 2012.[4,5] Laser, light, radiofrequency, and plasma technologies represent an important advance in skin rejuvenation in the options for patients. Physical, technological, and clinical research is currently carried out in order to optimize energy device–skin interaction and energy device efficacy-safety profile. The different energy device sources are further summarized following the different spectral features of the laser sources used:[6,7]

1. Ultraviolet (UV) laser and light sources: they are used primarily for the treatment of inflammatory skin diseases and/or vitiligo, as well as striae. The mechanism of action is immunomodulatory. The XeCl excimer laser emits at 308 nm, near the peak action spectrum for psoriasis. Other UV nonlaser sources such as the 355 nm have also been used for vitiligo and hypopigmentation disorders and various inflammatory diseases.
2. Violet intense pulsed light (IPL) spectra and low-power 410 nm LED and fluorescent lamps: both are used either alone or with aminolevulinic acid (ALA). Alone, the devices take advantage of endogenous porphyrins and kill *Propionibacterium acnes*. After application of ALA, this wavelength range is highly effective in creating singlet O_2 after absorption by PpIX.

Uses include treatment of actinic keratoses, actinic cheilitis, and basal cell carcinomas.
3. Near-infrared (IR)(A) (595, 755, and 810 nm): these wavelengths are used primarily to treat blood vessels and hyperpigmented lesions. They are positioned in the absorption spectrum for blood and melanin and will penetrate deeply enough to treat vessels up to 2 mm. Newer lasers, such as the pulsed-dye laser (595 nm), may be indicated for the treatment of port-wine stains and infantile hemangiomas. Q-switched lasers in this spectrum may be useful to treat multicolored tattoos.
4. Near-IR(B) 940 and 1064 nm: these two wavelengths have been used extensively for lager and deeper blood vessels on the legs and face. Because of the depth of penetration (on the order of millimeters), they are especially useful in coagulation of deeper blood vessels and selective follicle denaturation for safe and effective hair removal. Q-switched 1064 nm lasers are very effective on dark ink tattoos.
5. Medium-IR lasers (1320–1540 nm): they heat tissue water, shrink collagen, and are widely used in cosmetology for antiaging purposes, treatment of striae, and acne scarring (nonablative fractional procedures).
6. Far-IR systems: represented mainly by the CO_2 and Er:YAG lasers. Dermatologic applications are mainly surgical (warts, dermal nevi) and

cosmetological, thanks to their precision in ablation. Fractional CO_2 lasers guarantee a very precise epidermal and dermal heating that makes this device ideal for facial skin resurfacing (fine or moderate wrinkles, dyspigmentation, and acne scarring) on facial skin. Newer devices combine lasers to other energy sources such as radiofrequency in order to optimize antiaging dermatologic procedures.

7. Radiofrequency devices: as any form of energy, ablative or nonablative RF has the capacity to produce heat—and although each brandname application uses a slightly different technology, all work by resistive heating in the skin's deeper layers induce new collagen and elastin production and encourage cell turnover, helping skin become firmer, thicker, and more youthful looking.

8. Ultrasound devices: sound is defined as mechanical energy that spreads through a medium in the form of waves. During ultrasound procedures, there is typically a gel that is placed on top of the skin that allows the sound waves to be sent through the gel to target different areas of the body. Ultrasound sends off sound waves that can cause vibrations. Depending on the frequency, these vibrations create heat within the body that can be tailored for different effects in the skin: the stimulation of collagen or the breakdown of adipose tissue.

9. Plasma devices: plasma skin regeneration technology uses energy delivered from plasma rather than light or radiofrequency only. Plasma is typically generated by an energy discharge, which can include radiofrequency that causes ionization, excitation, or dissociation of gas or liquid molecules, leading to creation of various gaseous plasmas. The energy delivered produces a heating action that works at the skin's surface to remove old photo-damaged epidermal cells and below the skin surface or dermis to promote collagen growth.

OVERVIEW OF PROCEDURE-BASED TECHNOLOGY APPLICATIONS FOR ENERGY DEVICES

When considering the uses of energy-based devices, the most frequent patient requests are for skin rejuvenation including fine lines, wrinkles, pore size, acne, and acne scarring. The requests include an interest for an overall improvement in skin tone texture and color. The next 2 classes of treatment are where technology devices simulate or substitute for surgical procedures in that facial and neck contour improvement are sought such as reduction of jowls or submental fat. Lastly,

loose skin without fatty deposits may require skin tightening. These 3 categories are discussed later and various energy-based devices are listed and evaluated before analyzing issues such as Return on Investment (ROI) or costs of implementation. So the categories of clinical problems include those that include traditional skin rejuvenation objectives as well as the more recent advent of having technology devices simulate what was previously thought to be the domain of facial plastic surgery specifically correcting facial and neck contours as well as tightening loose skin. The latter 2 (contouring and skin tightening) applications became possible as treatment alternatives to face and neck lift surgery.

COSMETIC DERMATOLOGY APPLICATIONS

Many technology devices were developed to correct common skin problems, and the formation of early tech companies reflected a growing trend of patients to want options that addressed skin correction beyond what was typically available in the late nineteenth century such as skin care products and chemical peels. Problems such as vascularity and pigmentation as well as large pores and rhytids, acne, and acne scarring were approached by technology companies, and the initial production of lasers was collectively referred to as "Vascular & Pigmented" (IPL, Nd:YAG,KTP,Pulsed Dye et) lasers and those aimed at wrinkle reduction and "skin resurfacing" such as CO_2 and erbium. These devices were available in the early to mid-1990s, and in some cases development of vascular & pigmented lesion lasers were developed to treat dermatologic problems such as portwine stains or other hereditary pigmented disorders. As time has passed and with the growth of the aesthetic industry far more R&D has gone into primary aesthetic applications and less into "medically necessary" applications.

SKIN TIGHTENING

In 2004 Thermage (**Fig. 2**) was released and for the first time a technology device was released with the objective of addressing facial aging from a more comprehensive approach in treating overall laxity of the facial and head and neck skin and not simply addressing the appearance of skin. The method of action for Thermage was skin/dermal heating with the production of dermal collagen or "neocollagenesis" as the rejuvenative potential of the early thermal devices. Initially all skin tightening was viewed as a manifestation of increasing dermal collagen via thermal stimulation. The importance of the

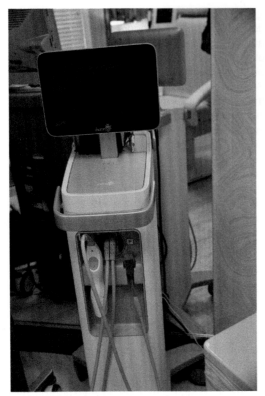

Fig. 2. Thermage has stood the test of time. Current Thermage FLX shown.

fibroseptal network (FSN) was not really addressed until later in that decade. Most of the limitations of transcutaneous devices centered around an inability to adequately treat/heat the skin without risking complications such as excess heat creating burns, hyper- or hypopigmentation, or contour irregularities due to localized fat ablation below the deep dermis. In 2007 the FDA approved the Smartlipo laser, which was initially positioned as a laser lipolysis device but was actually one of the first energy-based devices that had the potential to reduce fat, coagulate blood vessels and tighten collagen in the interstitial space. Before lasers leading the march to technology development for skin tightening including facial and neck contouring the only other class of device used "under the skin" was ultrasound technology, which was first described by Scuderi.[8]

CONTOURING OF SUBMENTUM AND JOWLS WITH FACIAL AND NECK SKIN TIGHTENING

From the early introduction of subdermal lasers (2007) for "fat reduction" it became clear that using subdermal devices was a way of doing augmented liposuction as a rejuvenative procedure of the face and neck. What I mean by this is Facial Plastic Surgeons would consider liposuction as a treatment modality for younger patients (**Fig. 3**) due to the intrinsic ability of younger skin to retract and not hang loosely after fat removal. The concern surgeons have is that a 50-year-old (**Fig. 4**) may not generate enough skin retraction and remodeling after fat removal/ablation and thus needs skin excision included as part of the rejuvenative procedure. The use of subdermal heating in fact makes liposuction a primary treatment modality for many of the older patients, as it creates a skin tightening process that in fact makes them react much as a younger patient due to the application of heat to the FSN. In 2007 we started treating the entire face and neck with subdermal laser energy. We reported this at the 2008 American Academy of Facial Plastic and Reconstructive Surgery meeting in Chicago, IL and at the ASLM [Aslms American Society For Laser Medicine And Surgery, Inc] meeting in 2009,[9] and the era of nonexcisional facial contouring with skin tightening was begun. These procedures generally include thermal ablation of the interstitial space (subcutaneous) followed by lipocontouring and then additional thermal treatment of the interstitial space for temperature-relevant endpoints now measured with thermal sensors. Recently we introduced a protocol for treating the deep subplatysmal space for additional contouring of the neck especially for the mandibular contour (**Fig. 5**). The treatment process and the development of an aesthetic laser, subspecialty of *subdermal laser surgery*, has developed over the past 12 years[10–12] and has been joined by many facial plastic surgeons and other aesthetic practitioners using devices that have been developed for the purpose of enhancing facial and neck contours with volume reduction combined with skin tightening.

EVALUATING TECHNOLOGY

I believe that deciding what technology you wish to explore requires deciding what your relationship to technology will be. Do you want to be a technology expert who is always on the forefront of new technologies or do you want to be more selective and invest in a select few devices that you think will be popular for your patients? Do you want to own something from each group we discussed earlier or just pick out the hot device? So, deciding on what your relationship to technology will be is important to think about because the investments are substantial and ongoing with maintenance contracts and other costs to operate. I think that

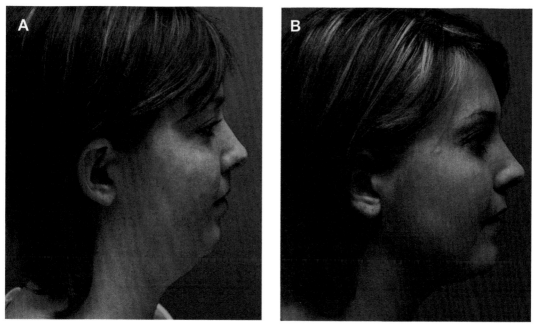

Fig. 3. A 26-year-old presented for lower face and neck sculpting. Shown before (*A*) and 4 months after (*B*) laser lipolysis with skin tightening.

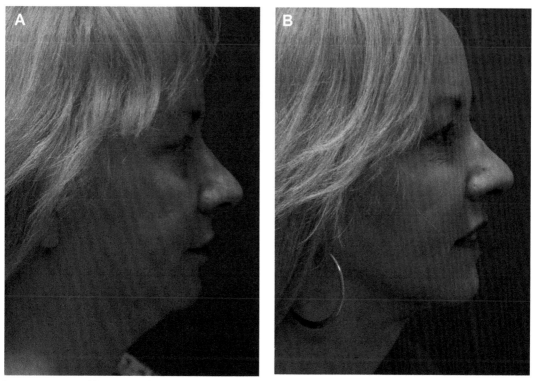

Fig. 4. A 58-year-old presents for facial rejuvenation. Treated with Renuvion interstitial facial sculpting. Shown before (*A*) and 4 months after operation (*B*).

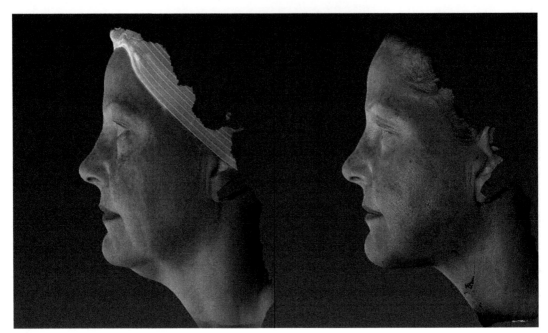

Fig. 5. A 58-year-old presenting for lower face and neck rejuvenation. Shown 1 week after minimally invasive neck lifting with deep cervicoplasty.

the day of not a few devices in the office have passed if you wish to practice facial plastic surgery including all aspects. This would not apply if you wish to be a superspecialist, say 90% rhinoplasty, in your practice. It is important to also consider to what extent you want to treat patients and if you are interested in a middle-of-the-road recovery or if you are willing to do completely ablative procedures that require considerable hand holding in the recovery process. That being said there is a benefit to looking at the workstation concept where multiple devices exist on one machine. This is particularly useful if you are going to hold maintenance contracts on them. One maintenance contract covering 3 devices is probably less expensive than covering 3 different devices. So, starting with a basic system, one offering 3 options, seems to be a good place to start. One being hair removal, one an IPL-based system, and one capable of more significant nonablative or mildly ablative skin rejuvenation. I think for those starting out with technology this is a test run and you can see how well things go with the implementation. Having the properly motivated and trained staff is also a very important necessity to consider. From a "spa type" investment you have to look at whether you want to proceed to facial contouring and skin tightening procedures. Today's technology also permits you to adopt hands-free lasers, cryolipolysis, or RF devices for noninvasive body contouring. When considering these investments,

you have to evaluate the current status of those devices in your direct market and whether you think the implementation will be successful. Talk to colleagues about their experience with the technology or device to get an idea if their acquisition was something they were pleased with. Longevity of technology has to be considered because if the latest greatest device suddenly is eclipsed by other technologies that are emerging you will hope that you will have the cost of the device recovered. Generally speaking, you should look for several procedures you can do with your technology if one of those goes cold. In the era of social media and plastic surgery blogs, read the patient reviews at the various review sites to see if high patient satisfaction is seen with the device you are contemplating. When looking at devices it will become apparent that there is a distribution of similar devices. Let us take RF microneedling as an example. There are many different options that work very similarly like the initial Infini (Lutronic) and Intensif (EndyMed) and newer options such as Morpheus 8 (InMode). Try to drill down on what is similar and what is different, for example, Profound (Syneron Candela) is very different than the ones mentioned earlier because it has temperature-controlled sensors in the needles. So, determine what type of the particular device type you are interested in in a technology sector. Many are the same, but some are not. So, examine the inner workings of the technology.

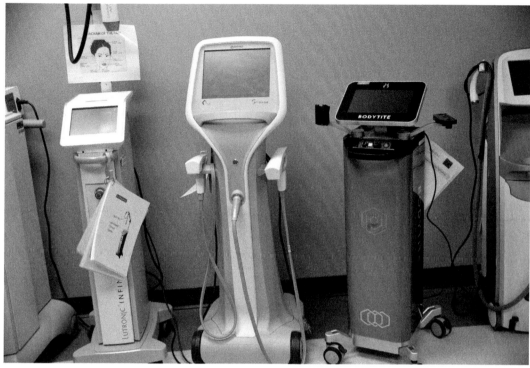

Fig. 6. Various microneedling options at our center. Each device has specific advantages and disadvantages. Shown are Infini, Morpheus 8, and Profound.

Another example for current contouring/skin tightening is laser versus RF versus plasma. So in looking at device capabilities you have to have a general idea of how the device works in order to competitively compare it with other devices.

FINANCIAL CONSIDERATIONS AND RETURN ON INVESTMENT

Technology devices can be insanely expensive to own and operate and so in the process of doing due diligence in exploring these devices you have to proceed slowly in evaluating the costs involved. Although "Return on Investment" is frequently mentioned, there is another ROI to be considered and that is "Return of Investment" or will I get the money invested back from the device I am considering. My personal approach to this is a bit different than most. As a technology expert I look at some of the investments as the cost of doing business and being able to have an in-depth experience with devices and technologies so that I can discuss them honestly with my colleagues who frequently call me for my opinions. I also want to maintain financial independence from the companies so that my opinions are genuine and not influenced by financial gain. This results in my having multiple devices

in the same technology format. For example, we have Infini, Morpheus 8, Fractora, and Profound, which are all RF microneedling devices (**Fig. 6**). Because I own and use them all I can give an unbiased opinion of the strengths and weaknesses of each device.

MARKETING AND PRACTICE POSITIONING

Because of the high cost of technology acquisition it is important to realize that promoting your newly acquired device is important for it to be successful. You should calculate this additional specific investment when considering the overall cost of the technology acquisition, and this includes marketing on your Website, internal and external marketing, and social media marketing. All of these are important to the successful implementation of new technology. Introductory discounts are important as well as device specific in office events to promote your new technology. I have been fortunate in that nearly all investments in my more than 30 devices I have not regretted and the objective here is to do your due diligence so that you will not regret the purchase especially if you are new to this technology "space".

SUMMARY

Aesthetic technology investments are becoming more necessary and common in establishing and developing a successful facial plastic surgery practice. The major concern about these investments are the high cost, concerns about longevity of technology, skilled personnel to operate the devices, and also concerns about the learning curve in achieving excellent long-term results, which translate to high patient satisfaction and increased patient to patient referrals. The technologies most relevant to facial plastic surgery practices include those typically associated with technology-based aesthetic technology practices including devices to treat vascular and pigmented lesions, acne and acne scarring, and rhytides. Recently the focus of technology has been on devices that help to contour and tighten the face and neck, including devices that are designed to tighten the FSN and create improvement in jowls and neck laxity without undergoing a full surgical procedure. When contemplating technology investments proper due diligence is required to learn about the specific technologies being considered as well as consulting with colleagues and patient sites on the Internet that evaluate patient satisfaction. Starting small in order to evaluate the success of implementation of new devices/technology is recommended as well as pursuing devices that can be used for more than one procedure.

REFERENCES

1. Feldman LS, Fuchshuber PR, Jones DB. The SAGES manual on the fundamental use of surgical energy (FUSE). Berlin/Heidelberg (Germany): Springer Science+Business Media, LLC; 2012.

2. Anderson RR, Parrish JA. Selective photothermolysis: precise microsurgery by selective absorption of pulsed radiation. Science 1983;220(4596):524–7.

3. Holcomb JD, Rousso KK, Rousso DE. Nitrogen plasma skin regeneration and aesthetic facial surgery. Multicenter Eval valuation of Concurrent Treatment. Arch Facial Plast Surg 2009;11(3):184–93.

4. Kilmer S, Shah SN, Fitzpatrick G, et al. A pilot study on the use of a plasma skin regeneration device (Portrait®PSR3) in full facial rejuvenation procedures. Lasers Med Sci 2007;22(2):101–9.

5. Gentile RD. Cool atmospheric plasma (J-plasma) and new options for facial contouring and skin rejuvenation of the heavy face and neck. Facial Plast Surg 2018;34(1):66–74.

6. Gentile RD. Renuvion/J-plasma for subdermal skin tightening facial contouring and skin rejuvenation of the face and neck. Facial Plast Surg Clin North Am 2019;27(3):273–90.

7. Nistico SP, Chiricozzi A, Tamburi F, et al. Lasers and energy devices for the skin: conventional and unconventional use. Biomed Res Int 2016;2016:9031091. Accessed June 1, 2019.

8. Scuderi N, De Vita R, D'Andrea F. Nouve prospettive nella liposuzione: La lipoemulsificazione. G Chir 1987;2:1–10.

9. Gentile RD. Smartlifting-A technological innovation for facial rejuvenation. Lasers Surg Med 2009;41(Supplement 21).

10. Gentile RD. SmartLifting fiber laser-assisted facial rejuvenation techniques. Facial Plast Surg Clin North Am 2011;19(02):371–87.

11. Gentile RD. Subcutaneous fiber laser and energy-based techniques for facial rejuvenation. In: Truswell WH, editor. Lasers and light, peels and abrasions. New York: Thieme Publishers; 2016. p. 47–74.

12. Gentile RD. Laser-assisted neck-lift: high-tech contouring and tightening. Facial Plast Surg 2011;27(4):331–45.

Psychiatric Disorders in Facial Plastic Surgery

Casper Candido (Capi) Wever, MD, PhD[a],*, Ana Maria Elisabeth (Anita) Wever, MSc[b], Mark Constantian, MD[c,d,1]

KEYWORDS

- Cosmetic surgery • Psychology • Borderline personality • Body dysmorphic syndrome

KEY POINTS

- Body dysmorphic disorder (BDD) and borderline personality disorder (BPD) are common in esthetic practices and may occur in up to 15% of patients.
- Although full-blown BDD and BPD may occur in a minority of esthetic patients, many more manifest traits that resemble these conditions.
- The likelihood of a satisfied surgical patient is exceedingly low in true BDD and BPD and surgery may worsen their premorbid condition.
- Avoiding surgery by adequate screening for BDD and BPD is hence essential.
- The standard of care for both conditions is a combination of cognitive behavioral therapy and selective serotonin reuptake inhibitor pharmacotherapy.

INTRODUCTION

Cosmetic facial surgery can provide satisfying results, and significantly improve self-confidence and self-esteem of patients, and most patients show little or no sign of psychological abnormality.[1–4] Yet facial surgery also potentially attracts individuals that can be difficult, if not impossible, to please. These cases have been subject of intense scrutiny for several decades.[5,6] Many of us have wondered over that singular case with a perfect postoperative result, yet who utterly failed to perceive this, and was moreover fully unresponsive to verbal intervention. What makes many patients happy with their surgical results, even if it is not spot-on at times, whereas others can engage in negative and even destructive behavior over a similar result? Understanding prevalent yet complex psychiatric disorders and their potential impact on patient behavior is quintessential in cosmetic facial surgery. In this review we discuss the global psychiatric context with a focus on two of the most prevalent and consequential conditions in the field: borderline personality disorder (BPD) and body dysmorphic disorder (BDD).[7]

SETTING THE STAGE: JUST UNHAPPY OR MENTAL DISORDER?

Every surgeon, and especially those that practice in hypercosmetic practices, will have to deal with patients that are not at the peak of happiness postsurgically. This is likely a source for stress, and may cause "blaming the patient" as a subliminal and unintended strategy.[7] Hence, one risk is that we unjustly label our dissatisfied patients as being psychological disturbed.

In rhinoplasty, the *a priori* likelihood of patients being unhappy is higher than in other cosmetic procedure.[8] The nature of the procedure makes that even small imperfections can have a meaningful esthetic impact. Also, to perform rhinoplasty to

[a] Department of Otolaryngology, Head & Neck Surgery, Leiden University Medical Center, Leiden, the Netherlands; [b] Chagalweg 18, Almere 1328 LE, the Netherlands; [c] Division of Plastic Surgery, Department of Surgery, University of Wisconsin School of Medicine and Public Health, Madison, WI, USA; [d] Department of Surgery, University of Virginia Medical School, Charlottesville, VA, USA
[1] Present address: 19 Tyler Street, Suite 302, Nashua, NH 03060-2979.
* Corresponding author. Benoordenhoutseweg 227-b, The Hague 2596 BE, the Netherlands.
E-mail address: capi.wever@xs4all.nl

Facial Plast Surg Clin N Am 28 (2020) 451–460
https://doi.org/10.1016/j.fsc.2020.06.003
1064-7406/20/© 2020 Elsevier Inc. All rights reserved.

comply with a high level of perfection is particularly difficult and requires experience and full dedication. Hence, the dissatisfied rhinoplasty patient needs not be "mad." Rather the hypercosmetic patient, the patient who is generally pretty and desires perfecting of her looks, places surgeons for the colossal challenge of improving on an already beautiful face.[1,8] Social media and the rage of selfies has complicated this problem even more, and may have created a level of expectation that one simply cannot realistically deliver on at a reliable rate.[9] Indeed early studies revealed that technical-surgical failure to achieve perfection was the most common cause of patient dissatisfaction, rather than any kind of disorder.[10,11] Given the high expectations of our times, it is unlikely that the extremely high satisfaction rates reported in the 1960s can be replicated in our modern times.[12] Hence one early question we should ask ourselves is if we achieved a realistically satisfactory result.

Another issue that may play a role is the potentially type-changing nature of cosmetic surgery.[5] Indeed, rhinoplasty in particular can change the Gestalt of patients. An extreme type-changing procedure may require adaptation time, even if the esthetic result is otherwise flawless. Shridharani and coworkers[13] have referred to this as a "loss of identity syndrome." Ethnic issues may play a compounding role here, because some ethnicities perceive specific facial features as intrinsic.[14] Hence a second question we should ask ourselves is if we type-changed an unhappy patient too much, or perhaps too little.

Yet in understanding pathology as underlying dissatisfaction, the focus ought not so much be on dissatisfaction itself but rather on behavior, which is a critical distinction. After all, even if surgical results are suboptimal not all patients respond negatively. Although only few are truly happy, and many may experience different levels of distress, most are at least collected in their response. It is the immature response to an optimal or suboptimal surgical response that separates patients with a potential troublesome personality structure from those that are just unhappy. It is a key to identifying genuine personality disorders.

PERSONALITY DISORDERS

Rather than viewing personality disorders as a unique and distinct category, they should be perceived on a gliding scale of human personality traits that are common yet variable in intensity. Hence all people have specific personality traits that may more or less identify who they are, but they typically do not interfere with normal functioning. Yet when these traits scale-up they may well start inhibiting us from leading a full and satisfying life. It is under such circumstances that we consider personality "disorders" rather than just "traits." Personality disorders are, hence, like a blowup version of normalcy.

Personality disorders are common, affecting about 10% of the population. They usually have an onset in adolescence or early adulthood and are divided in three clusters. Cluster A disorders include paranoid personality disorder, and are unlikely to present themselves with an esthetic need. Cluster B personality disorders include BPD and narcissistic personality disorder, and are likely fairly common in those seeking cosmetic surgery. Cluster C includes avoidant personality, obsessive-compulsive personality, and depended personality. BDD, however, is categorized under the obsessive compulsive disorder (OCD) and related disorders and not under Cluster C personality disorder. Yet it is highly relevant for cosmetic medicine and is also discussed here.

BORDERLINE PERSONALITY DISORDER

The pathogenesis of BPD is multifold and has a strong genetic foundation. In terms of psychodynamic cause, several pathways have been highlighted, among which is childhood trauma.[15] The onset of BPD is typically in adolescence and progresses with age. The prevalence in the general population is around 2%, with females being more frequently affected.[4] In a cosmetic environment the rate of occurrence has been found to be much higher, some reporting almost 1 in 10.[16] Morioka and Ohkubo[4] suggest that BPD patients consult for cosmetic surgery through two general pathways. The first is the route of self-injury. The second is the route of insatiable requests for cosmetic procedures, based on their chronic unstable identity and a desire to maintain the relationship with their surgeon. Hence many so-called "polysurgery addicts" are believed to suffer from BPD.[4]

People with BPD suffer from fear of abandonment or separation insecurity, unstable emotions, anxiousness, depressiveness, unstable and conflicted close relationships, unstable identities, and unstable self-direction.[17,18] In addition they tend to be impulsive and engage in risk-taking behavior, in self-destructive or self-harm behavior, and can sometimes manifest paranoid thoughts. People who suffer from BPD are prone to external splitting, which means that those around them are categorized along a strict line of good versus bad. Those that abandon them or threaten to, may instantly flip from being a hero to a villain. Similarly, internal splitting also occurs. It is suggested that when BPD patients go through a phase of perceiving themselves as "bad," impulsive self-harm may occur. Self-inflicted cuts or burns to the arms or legs are common: some authors report comorbid BPD in more than 50% of self-muti-lants.[19] Multiple tattoos or piercings can also be an expression of self-injury. Ultimately, suicide-attempts are more prevalent among people with BPD, completed suicide being reported in up to 10%.[4,20]

BPD commonly coexists with other mental conditions. It can, for example, manifest itself in similar terms as classic mood disorders, such as depression and bipolar disorder, and may cluster around several supplementary personality disorders, such as avoidant and dependent personality disorder.[4] Especially bipolar disease can coexist, because BPD patients are equally inclined toward impulsivity and consequent emotional instability. There also seems to be a significant overlap with eating disorders, with 10% to 15% of BDD patients having comorbid BPD.[21] Morioka and Ohkubo[4] suggest that surgeons should look for the warning signs shown in **Box 1**.

People with BPD are poor candidates for cosmetic procedures, because their outcome is usually disappointing and troublesome.[4,22] Moreover external splitting can eventually turn their disappointment toward the treatment team. Lawsuits and even violence have been reported.[16] Standard of care consists of psychotherapy, and may include pharmacotherapy.[23] In terms of how to handle patients with BPD, Morioka and Ohkubo[4] suggest "a flexible and individualized approach and confident attitude." Given their sensitivity for impending abandonment,

maintaining a positive relationship is key. At the same time, drawing clear boundaries is also of importance. Hence one ought to be analytical and detailed about the expected benefits and confident in the treatment plan, because patients themselves are lacking in this respect. Smaller procedures are a way to divert attention away, toward a less risky treatment plan.

Protecting the team's resilience if trouble does occur is imperative. Experiencing a BPD patient in a downward spiral can deeply erode the morale of the treating team. Those that provide care for BPD patients are at high risk for burnout.[24] Discussing the case regularly in team meetings, and agreeing on a single person to communicate with the patient on a day-to-day basis are general pearls that are of help.

BODY DYSMORPHIC DISORDER

BDD is likely the most prevalent of mental disorders in terms of its relevance to cosmetic surgery. It was first described in the late 1960s, even though related concepts emerged in medical literature more than a century ago as "dysmorphophobia."[25–27] The formal diagnosis was established in Diagnostic and Statistical Manual of Mental Disorders (DSM)-3, separating delusional and nondelusional variants as separate entities.

BDD is defined as a disproportional obsession with a minimal or imagined defect of the body, where the disproportionality relates to its obsessive undertone and dysfunctional embedding. In the historic diagnosis of dysmorphophobia, this has been described as an obsessive thought of being ugly, later described as imagined ugliness.[25,28] The likelihood of being satisfied with cosmetic surgery is exceedingly low, leading to insatiable sequential request for sequential procedures.[26] In DSM-5 BDD is categorized under OCD and related disorders, as a specific variant of OCD. Delusional and nondelusional variants are nowadays viewed as expressions of the same disease.

The population incidence of BDD has been found to be around 1.5 to 2.5 in 100, and it affects both genders about equally. Yet in those that seek cosmetic procedures, the incidence has been found to be significantly higher.[13,29–32] Sarwer reports a prevalence of 7% in women seeking cosmetic surgery, whereas Veale reports almost double that number.[33–36] Self-referrals may be for cosmetic surgery, injectables, but also for dermatology and dentistry. Obsessive attention to body muscle mass (muscle dysmorphia) may also be a variant of BDD.[37] The condition is typically chronic and rarely leads to remission.

Box 1
Warning signs of BPD

- Female gender
- Early 20s to 30s
- History of psychiatric disorders
- History of adverse events in childhood
- History of multiple cosmetic procedures
- Dissatisfaction or anger toward previous surgeon
- Self-harm behavior, multiple tattoos and/or piercings
- Splitting behavior
- Psychosocial impairment
- Concern with one or more body parts

More than 80% of cosmetic surgeons are said to have operated on patients who, in hindsight, probably had BDD.[38] These cases were mostly unknown to psychological services.[9] Cosmetic rhinoplasty is the single procedure that BDD cases are most likely to request, and the onset of BDD and the desire for rhinoplasty tend to overlap in late adolescence.[39] Although these patients may behave maturely at their consultation, things can drastically and rapidly change postsurgically.[15]

Hence, what characterizes BDD is the severe discordance between the emotional attribution to a specific facial shape, versus what others perceive. Indeed Edgerton and coworkers[40] included the degree to which the surgeon can empathize with the patient's desire as a key indicator. Hence, there is a severe and intrusive preoccupation with a physical shape that is imagined or hardly perceivable, and this concern is causing significant distress and, critically, impairs normal functioning. For up to 40% this belief is actively delusional, implying that correction is impossible, and there is a lack of disease insight.[41] Most, however, suffer from what is referred to as "overvalued ideas" rather than true delusion.[42] Although a small minority of cases may meet the full criteria, more than 40% of cosmetic rhinoplasty cases may have some symptoms of BDD.[26,43]

One of the problems with BDD is the lack of an unambiguous diagnostic tool, and the sensitivity to social and cultural vignettes. Researchers may hold preconceptual views of cosmetic surgery as cultural victimization, which may bias their definitions.[36,37,44,45] What exactly comprises a preoccupation with a perceived defect is ultimately not a matter of science. For example, all surgeons that work in a cosmetic practice know that many, if not most, of our clients are skewed toward being preoccupied with their appearance, and are detailed in their judgment. Some have argued that to avoid such bias, the nature or assumed severity of the facial trait should not even matter, but rather the emotional attribution to that trait. Hence, in this respect BDD is more one end of a spectrum rather than a unique entity. Although popular media and some sciences may implore on BDD as a construct, blaming unrealistic cultural standards and social media, true BDD does occur. The defining trait that sets BDD apart from subclinical obsession with one's appearance is dysfunction.

Hence, what sets people with true BDD apart is dysfunction. They pervasively think about their face for hours at a time, averaging 3 to 8 hours per day.[41] They are overwhelmed with distressing thoughts about their appearance; have low self-esteem as a consequence; engage in compulsive rituals, such as mirror-gazing; and are inhibited to function normally.[26] They may avoid people or skip school or work, out of shame, and hence disfunction psychosocially. BDD patients believe they are worthless and the constant subject of mockery.

In a clinical setting BDD patients are extremely detailed about their esthetic concerns, sometimes leading to drawings and self-morphed pictures, and even proto-professionalizing behavior where they suggest which surgical technique to undertake. However, they also tend to be secretive about their concerns because they fear social reprimanding. In a clinical setting they may also fear not being operated on if disclosing their condition (**Box 2**).

Full-blown cases of BDD are unlikely to be encountered in cosmetic practices, because these individuals are unlikely to be functional enough to make their way to the office. So, this correction needs to be taken into consideration when interpreting the DSM definition of BDD, which may be skewed toward overt dysfunctional psychiatry. The patients that cosmetic surgeons see are not the housebound, delusional individuals described in the mental health literature. Instead, surgeons meet apparently functional, often highly performing people seeking surgery, or more surgery. Thus, a way of understanding and recognizing these patients, a method of defining surgical BDD, would be useful in patient selection and safety.

Even for dedicated researchers, the cause BDD has been elusive. Neurobiologic processing issues may coexplain why BDD patients attribute such disproportional values to a specific facial shape. It has indeed been suggested through functional MRI studies that BDD patients process visual memory differently, lacking in global memory and focusing on detailed visual cues instead.[46] Structural differences at serotonin and dopamine levels have also been implicated.[47–49] A genetic trend

---

Box 2
BDD criteria (DSM-5)

- Preoccupation with one or more perceived defect or flaws in physical appearance that are not observable or seem slight to others

- Repetitive behavior (eg, mirror checking) or mental acts (eg, rumination) in response to these concerns

- Preoccupation causing clinically significant distress or impairment in functioning

- Preoccupation not explained by eating disorder, and not about bodyfat

has been reported, because 5% to 20% of BDD subject have a first-degree family member also suffering from the condition.[39,50] A genetic relation with OCD has also been reported.[48,50]

Yet environmental or sociodynamic explanations also apply.[26] Social environment can, it is assumed, modify or reaffirm the negative emotional attribution to a specific facial shape. The family is an important modifier in this context, explaining why part of the BDD literature focusses on family environment. A negative family environment, where the child is rejected, based on appearance in particular, is believed to play a causative role, particularly during adolescence.[51] Constantian[15] and others have related BDD to childhood trauma and regressed states. The sense of being defective is being localized in childhood, through a series of distinct pathways, eventually leading to body shame, which connects low self-esteem to body shape and can lead people to inappropriately seek out plastic surgery. The common denominator is that a child is given the feeling of not being good enough or fit for his or her parents.

In more than 90% BDD coincides with other and multiple psychiatric conditions, such as depression, anxiety, social phobia, OCD, and eating disorders.[52] Some studies found that more than 50% of BDD patients have a lifetime history of anxiety.[39] Personality disorders are common, mostly Cluster C. This implies that a history of psychiatric comorbidity may be viewed to strengthen the clinical case for BDD. A repeat history of cosmetic procedures, revision cases that started their primary rhinoplasty with a near-normal nose, and cases that present themselves as depressed and highly demanding are perhaps at higher risk of BDD.[14] Personality disorders overlap in terms of definition, and commonly coexist with each other or other psychological problems, such as depression or anxiety, making diagnosing and managing these cases a complex task. BDD patients, for example, commonly manifest the same splitting behavior as is common in BPD. The two commonly coexist and may overlap.

The typical presentation of the BDD patient preoperatively has been laid out. Yet if one operates on these cases, knowingly or unknowingly, the course is typically one of intense and unmitigated dissatisfaction with the results, in spite of possible initial satisfaction at cast removal. Surgery is hence not an adequate nor suitable solution for these people's grievances, because only in a minority it leads to remission. In some cases it may even worsen the condition.[37,53] Constantian and Lin[54] report only 3% of BDD cases being happy with their result after a single rhinoplasty

procedure, typically leading to an insatiable need for sequential procedures. Patients are typically inaccessible for argument, angry, and can spin into fierce aggression and sometimes social isolation. Aggression can express itself physically, but also legally or, nowadays, though social media. Several cases of aggression toward surgeons have been reported. Hence, their unhappiness deeply intertwines with negative affect toward the operating surgeon. Feeling betrayed, which may reveal coinciding of BPD, is a key emotion that is described repeatedly.[14] Aggression can also turn on oneself, because the annual rate of completed suicide is more than 40 times that of normal population.[41]

Given the potential impact on the postoperative course, timely diagnosing BDD at the intake procedure is appropriate. However, the diagnosis is commonly missed.[37,41] Phillips and Hollander[41] recommend screening for BDD in cosmetic surgery. Several tools stand at our disposition for this purpose. Some are based on experience, and specific red flags can be probed for during the consultation intake. Additionally, a specific number of questionnaires has been developed, specifically the Body Dysmorphic Disorder Examination Self-Report[55] and the Yale-Brown Obsessive Compulsive Scale for Body Dysmorphic Disorder.[56] Yet psychological questionnaires, be it disease specific or generic, alone cannot solve the dilemma of screening for psychologically complicated patients.[14] Although BPD and BDD patients are likely to fall through the cracks, many more may suffer from a range of emotional distress unrelated to their surgical desire. For others, emotional distress may be an adequate response. Many patients resist the diagnosis, if only because it precludes surgery. Hence some commonsensical perspective remains useful. Some practical signs that notify of impending problems are shown in **Box 3**.[9,41]

The gold standard of management of BDD is treatment with a selective serotonin reuptake inhibitor–type antidepressant in a high dose, reducing distress in up to almost three-quarters of cases. Referral for cognitive behavioral therapy and, if trauma related, EMDR therapy, is a good adjunct therapy.[37,39,57–60] Pharmacotherapy is especially essential for more severe cases of BDD, and undertreatment is common.[41]

FAMILY HISTORY AND CHILDHOOD TRAUMA AS A COMMON PATHWAY

About 20 years ago physicians at Kaiser Permanente in San Diego, California devised a weight loss program that seemed to have infinite promise.

The program was a failure. Instead of thin, happy people, the program generated depression, divorce, anxiety attacks, and suicide attempts. Many patients regained their lost weight. The researchers also uncovered the disturbing fact that behind the medicating effect of overeating were stories of childhood abuse and neglect. They reluctantly concluded that obesity was not a problem for these patients, but rather a solution.[61] Compelled to look further, Drs Vincent Felitti and Robert Anda studied the types of childhood trauma they were seeing, releasing their findings in 17,337 patients. When this middle class (80% White, 10% Black, 10% Asian) general medical population was asked about 10 common types of childhood abuse or neglect (emotional abuse, emotional neglect, physical abuse, physical neglect, sexual abuse, violence against the mother, divorce, alcohol or drug abuse in the family, mental illness in the family, imprisonment, or suicide), 64% had at least one positive answer. Furthermore, the more positive answers patients had, the worse their health: heart disease, pulmonary disease, hypertension, hypercholesterolemia, depression, obesity, and many other common adult illnesses.[62–65]

Constantian's Adverse Childhood Experiences Study (ACE) duplicated the study in a plastic and reconstructive surgery population. Only postoperative patients were tested, putting results in context. Was patient behavior depressed? How much pain medication did they need? Did the patients mention shame? What were their current health problems? Most importantly, were the patients satisfied postoperatively? Patients younger than age 21 were excluded. Participation was explicitly voluntary, but not one patient refused to be included. Two hundred-eighteen patients completed the survey, 76% women and 34% men. Ninety-four percent of the patients were White, 2% Black, 2% Asian, and 2% Latino. Mean age was 54 (range, 22–81). Seventy-nine percent had completed college or graduate school. Seventy-eight percent were employed, 10% unemployed, and 12% retired. Of the entire group, 86% were esthetic surgery patients (80% rhinoplasty and 20% other facial surgery or breast surgery) and 14% were reconstructive patients (skin cancers, reconstructive facial surgery, or hand surgery). Most patients had health insurance or income that covered esthetic surgery. The study population shared similarities to the Kaiser group and was not disadvantaged.

Among the rhinoplasty patients, 33% were primary rhinoplasties and 67% were revision patients. Seventy-five percent of the revision patients originally had normal noses. Typical expressed reasons for having had surgery were: "to be as pretty as my sister," "because I was an ugly baby," "so people would love me" (**Table 1**).

Whereas 64% of the Kaiser patients had at least one positive answer, 79% of this study's patients did (*P*<.001). Reconstructive patients had almost the same individual positive scores as the Kaiser patients (61% vs 64%, respectively). Not only were overall prevalences higher than the Kaiser group, but 4 of the 10 individual trauma types

---

Box 3
Practical warning signs

- Disconnect between intensity of preoccupation and severity of problem
- Impairment in normal socioemotional functioning (ie, school, work, and relations)
- Preoccupation (>1 hour per day) with appearance (ie, mirror gazing, camouflaging)
- Referential thinking (that others also perceive the problem as intensely)
- Previous requests for surgery
- Unrealistic expectations
- Demanding or unpleasant behavior toward personnel
- Viewing surgery as the solution to problems in other domains of life

---

Table 1
Component rates for ACE patients

	Our Patients (%)	Kaiser Value (%)	*P* value
Emotional abuse	41	11	<.0001
Physical abuse	25	28	.824
Sexual abuse	23	21	.184
Emotional neglect	38	15	<.0001
Physical neglect	12	9	.132
Parental separation or divorce	28	23	.082
Mother treated violently	11	13	.742
Household substance abuse	36	27	.002
Household mental illness	29	19	<.0001
Incarcerated household member	6	5	.149

were significantly higher than the Kaiser Permanente group (emotional abuse, emotional neglect, household substance abuse, and household mental illness). Separating the study groups according to their reasons for surgery, revealing differences were found. The mean ACE score for reconstructive patients was 2.0 but for BDD patients it was 4.3 (P<.029). Similarly, whereas 12.5% of the Kaiser patients had a total of ACE of four or more, similar to our reconstructive patients (16%), BDD groups had more than double the Kaiser rate at 36%. Like the Kaiser Permanente study, the number of positive ACE answers correlated with patient health. Even in this small population, dose-related correlations existed with depression, hypertension, hyperlipidemia, obesity, headaches, cancer, recreational drug use, irritable bowel, asthma, chronic obstructive pulmonary disease, arthritis, and excessive requests for pain medication.

This patient population, with an average age of 56, had health problems that correlated with their childhood trauma and manifested 35 to 50 years later. For many individuals, the effects of childhood do not dissipate: their minds, behaviors, lifestyles, and abilities to care for themselves each suffer. Detailed data are beyond the scope of this article but will be published shortly.[14] However, when segregating the groups according to surgical type (reconstructive, cosmetic nonrhinoplasty, primary rhinoplasty, revision patients who originally had deformities, and revision patients who originally had normal noses), those who originally had normal noses were youngest at their first surgeries, youngest at their first other cosmetic surgeries, most likely to be single (55%), and the most likely to explicitly mention shame to the surgeon (73% compared with 16% of reconstructive patients, 24% of cosmetic non-rhinoplasty patients, 39% of primary patients, and 64% of other revision rhinoplasty patients; P<.001).

Childhood abuse and neglect create shame, most commonly body shame.[66] If we begin with self-injurious, obsessive, intemperate, poor adult health, or addictive behaviors including BDD and work backward, each leads to dysfunctional family systems, shame, and childhood neglect or abuse, independent of socioeconomic conditions.[67–69] If we begin with childhood, the effects of developmental trauma can produce body shame-based, self-injurious, obsessive, intemperate, or addictive behaviors; poor adult health; and BDD.[66] Thus the connection between family, childhood, body shame, and body image disorders works in either direction, starting from childhood or starting from its adult sequelae. Adding our observations to the existing literature, it is possible to trace a pathway in which childhood trauma is the seed; shame its core manifestation; and dysregulation, addictions, and disease are its poisonous blooms. Many elective plastic surgery patients have had traumatic childhoods that impact self-worth and that can later manifest as body shame, perfectionism, an obsessive desire for plastic surgery, or postoperative anger, even with good results. The often inexplicable and sometimes irrational behavior that so taxes theses patients' families, friends, and caregivers is not their fault.

Thus, surgical BDD is not determined by what happens after surgery, but what goes before. Not every unhappy patient is body dysmorphic. Postoperative distress is not the key. The key to surgical BDD is what drove the surgery: shame and the desire for self worth. These patients cited original motives of self-esteem, self-perfection, or shame, not deformity. Any addictive substance, not even repeated plastic surgery, will never be enough to satisfy the patient's goal. That is why the size of the deformity does not justify the patient's level of distress. Why should it? It is not about the deformity.

DISCUSSION

The general population incidence of mental illness is estimated to be around 20%. Among clients that visit for cosmetic surgery, however, the incidence is believed to be significantly higher, some reporting half or even more meeting International Statistical Classification of Diseases and Related Health Problems-10 criteria for mental disorder.[16] In general the estimate of the incidence of psychopathology in patients seeking cosmetic surgery has been highest in earlier reports (1950s and 1960s) and has shown a consistently decreasing trend over time, perhaps suggesting a role of cultural vignettes.[26] Mental disease in itself is not by definition a reason to avoid cosmetic surgery, because many have been shown to be satisfied with the results of surgery.[40] It is those, however, that are unlikely to be happy regardless of the surgical results, and those that are at risk to harm themselves or the treatment team, that need to be identified. BPD and BDD are the two most relevant to cosmetic surgery. Both conditions occur in about 10% to 15% of cosmetic candidates and tend to coexist with other mental disorders. BPD and BDD patients are considered poor candidates for surgery because the likelihood of aggravating their premorbid condition is high and the likelihood for a satisfying outcome low. Adequate screening for these conditions is hence considered critical, even though milder cases may be able to dodge these instruments. Pragmatic vigilance for mental comorbidity, social dysfunction, and childhood trauma may hence be of use.

DISCLOSURE

None.

REFERENCES

1. Groenman NH, Sauer HC. Personality characteristics of cosmetic surgical insatiable patients. Psychother Psychosom 1983;40(1-4):241–5.
2. Litner -JA, Rotenberg-BW, Dennis -M, et al. Impact of cosmetic facial surgery on satisfaction with appearance and quality of life. Arch Facial Plast Surg 2008;10(2):79–83.
3. Honigman RJ, Phillips KA, Castle DJ. A review of psychosocial outcomes for patients seeking cosmetic surgery. Plast Reconstr Surg 2004; 113(4):1229–37.
4. Morioka D, Ohkubo F. Borderline personality disorder and aesthetic plastic surgery. Aesthetic Plast Surg 2014;38(6):1169–76.
5. Goin J, Goin M. Changing the body: psychological effects of plastic surgery. Williams and Wilkins; 1981.
6. Edgerton MT, Langman MW, Pruzinsky T. Patients seeking symmetrical recontouring for "perceived" deformities in the width of the face and skull. Aesthetic Plast Surg 1990;14(1):59–73.
7. Herruer JM, Prins JB, Heerbeek N, et al. Negative predictors for satisfaction in patients seeking facial cosmetic surgery: a systematic review. Plast Reconstr Surg 2015;135(6):1596–605.
8. Slator R, Harris DL. Are rhinoplasty patient potentially mad? Br J Plast Surg 1992;45(4):307–10.
9. Sweis IE, Spitz J, Barry DR, et al. A review of body dysmorphic disorder in aesthetic surgery patients and the legal implications. Aesthetic Plast Surg 2017;41(4):949–54.
10. Jacobson WE, Edgerton MT, Meyer E, et al. Psychiatric evaluation of male patients seeking cosmetic surgery. Plast Reconstr Surg 1960;26:356–72.
11. Meyer E, et al. Motivational patterns in patients seeking elective cosmetic surgery. Psychosom Med 1960;22:193–201.
12. Neaman KC, Boettcher AK, Do -VH, et al. Cosmetic rhinoplasty: revision rates revisited. Aesthet Surg J 2013;33(1):31–7.
13. Shridharani SM, Magarakis M, Manson PN, et al. Psychology of plastic and reconstructive surgery: a systematic clinical review. Plast Reconstr Surg 2010;126(6):2243–51.
14. Constantian MB, Hein R, Zaborek N. Prevalence of adverse childhood experiences in plastic surgery patients: towards a definition of "surgical body dysmorphic disorder". PRS, in press.
15. Constantian MB. Childhood abuse, body shame, and addictive plastic surgery. New Your: Routledge; 2018.
16. Napoleon A. The presentation of personalities in plastic surgery. Ann Plast Surg 1993;31(3):193–208.
17. Kornhaber R, Haik J, Sayers J, et al. People with borderline personality disorder and burns: some considerations for health professionals. Issues Ment Health Nurs 2017;38(9):767–8.
18. American Psychiatric Association. Desk reference to the diagnostic criteria from DSM-5. American Psychiatric Publishing; 2013. p. 93–114.
19. Nock MK, Joiner TE, Gordon KH, et al. Non-suicidal self-injury among adolescents: diagnostic correlates and relation to suicide attempts. Psychiatry Res 2006;144(1):65–72.
20. Leichsenring F, Leibling E, Kruse J, et al. Borderline personality disorder. Lancet 2011;377(9759):74–84.
21. Bjornsson AS, Didie ER, Grant JE, et al. Age at onset and clinical correlates in body dysmorphic disorder. Compr Psychiatry 2013;54-(7):893–903.
22. Bowyer L, Krebs G, Mataix-Cols D, et al. A critical review of cosmetic treatment outcomes in body dysmorphic disorder. Body Image 2016;19:1–8.
23. Grant BF, Chou SP, Goldstein RB, et al. Prevalence, correlates, disability, and comorbidity of DSM-IV borderline personality disorder: results from the wave 2 national epidemiologic survey on alcohol and related disorders. J Clin Psychiatry 2008; 69(4):533–45.
24. Mortimer-Jones S, Morrison P, Munib A, et al. Recovery and borderline personality disorder: a description of the innovative open borders program. Issues Ment Health Nurs 2016;37(9):624–30.
25. Morselli E. La psichiatria moderna nei suoi rapport con le alter scienze. Naples: 1891.
26. Crerand CE, Franklin ME, Sarwer DB. Body dysmorphic disorder and cosmetic surgery. Plast Reconstr Surg 2006;118(7):167e–80e.
27. Varma A, Rastogi R. Recognizing body dysmorphic disorder (dysmorphophobia). J Cutan Aesthet Surg 2015;8(3):165–8.
28. Higgins S, Wysong A. Cosmetic surgery and body dysmorphic disorder: an update. Int J Womens Dermatol 2017;4(1):43–8.
29. Wilson JB, Arprey CJ. Body dysmorphic disorder: suggestions for detection and treatment in a surgical dermatology practice. Dermatol Surg 2004;30(11): 1391–9.
30. Sarwer DB, Wadden TA, Pertschuk MJ, et al. The psychology of cosmetic surgery: a review and conceptualization. Clin Psychol Rev 1998;18(1):1–22.
31. Andreasen NC, Bardach J. Dysmorphophobia: symptom or disease? Am J Psychiatry 1977; 134(6):673–6.

32. Veale D, Gledhill LJ, Christodoulou P, et al. Body dysmorphic disorder in different settings: a systematic review and estimated weighted prevalence. Body Image 2016;18:168–86.

33. Picavet V, Gabriels L, Jorissen M, et al. Screening tools for body dysmorphic disorder in a cosmetic surgery setting. Laryngoscope 2011;121(12): 2535–41.

34. Pavan C, Simonato P, Marini M, et al. Psychopathologic aspects of body dysmorphic disorder: a literature review. Aesthetic Plast Surg 2008;32(3):473–84.

35. Vulink NC, Sigurdsson V, Kon M, et al. Body dysmorphic disorder in 3-8% of patients in outpatient dermatology and plastic surgery clinics. Ned Tijdschr Geneeskd 2006;150-2:97–100.

36. Sarwer DB. Body image in cosmetic surgical and dermatological practice. In: Castle DJ, Phillips KA, editors. Disorders of body image. Petersfield; 2002.

37. Tod D, Edwards C, Cranswick I. Muscle dysmorphia: current insights. Psychol Res Behav Manag 2016; 3(9):179–88.

38. Sarwer DB, Spitzer -JC. Body image dysmorphic disorder in persons who undergo aesthetic medical treatments. Aesthet Surg J 2012;32:999–1009.

39. Phillips KA. The broken mirror: understanding and treating body dysmorphic disorder. Revised and expanded edition. New York: Oxford University Press; 2005.

40. Edgerton MT, Langman MW, Pruzinsky T. Plastic surgery and psychotherapy in 100 psychologically disturbed patients. Plast Reconstr Surg 1991;88(4): 594–608.

41. Phillips KA, Hollander E. Treating body dysmorphic disorder with medication: evidence, misconceptions, and a suggested approach. Body Image 2008;5(1):13–27.

42. Laugharne R, et al. Dysmorphophobia by proxy. J R Soc Med 1997;90:266

43. Picavet VA, Gabriels L, Grietens J, et al. Preoperative symptoms of body dysmorphic disorder determine postoperative satisfaction and quality of life in aesthetic rhinoplasty. Plast Reconstr Surg 2013; 131(4):861–8.

44. Abbas OL, Karadavut U. Analysis of the factors affecting men's attitudes towards cosmetic surgery: body image, media exposure, social network use, masculine gender role stress and religious attitudes. Aesthetic Plast Surg 2017;41(6):1454–62.

45. Sarcu D, Adamson P. Psychology of the facelift patient. Facial Plast Surg 2017;33(3):252–9.

46. Deckersbach T, Savage CR, Phillips KA, et al. Characteristics of memory disfunction in body dysmorphic syndrome. J Int Neuropsychol Soc 2000;6(6): 673–81.

47. Marazziti D, Dell'Osso L, Presta S. Platelet [3H]paroxetine binding in patients with OCD-related disorders. Psychiatry Res 1999;89(3):223–8.

48. Monzani B, Rijsdijk F, Iervolino AC, et al. Evidence for a genetic overlap between body dysmorphic concerns and obsessive-compulsive symptoms in an adult female community twin sample. Am J Med Genet B Neuropsychiatr Genet 2012;159B(4):376–82.

49. Gabbay V, O'Dowd MA, Weiss AJ, et al. Body dysmorphic disorder triggered by medical illness. Am J Psychiatry 2002;159(3):492.

50. Bienvenu O, Samuels J, Riddle M, et al. The relationship of obsessive-compulsive disorder to possible spectrum disorders: results from a family study. Biol Psychiatry 2000;48(4):287–93.

51. Phillips KA. Body dysmorphic disorder: diagnosis and treatment of imagined ugliness. J Clin Psychiatry 1996;57(suppl 8):61–4.

52. Hundscheid T, van der Hulst RR, Rutten BP, et al. Stoornis in de lichaamsbeleving bij patienten binnen de cosmetische chirurgie. Tijdschr Psychiatr 2014; 56(8):514–22.

53. Philips KA, McElroy SL. Insight, overvalued ideation, and delusional thinking in body dysmorphic disorder: theoretical and treatment implications. J Nerv Ment Dis 1993;181(11):699–702.

54. Constantian MB, Lin CP. Why some patients are unhappy: part 2. relationship of nasal shape and trauma history to surgical success. Plast Reconstr Surg 2014;134(4):836–51.

55. Rosen JC, Reiter J. Development of the body dysmorphic disorder examination. Behav Res Ther 1996;34(9):755–66.

56. Phillips KA, Hollander E, Rasmussen SA, et al. A severity rating scale for body dysmorphic disorder. Psychopharmacol Bull 1997;33(1):17–22.

57. Allen LA, Woolfolk RL. Cognitive behavioral therapy for somatoform disorders. Psychiatr Clin North Am 2010;33(3):579–93.

58. Philips KA, Albertini RS, Rasmussen SA. A randomized placebo-controlled trial of fluoxetine in body dysmorphic syndrome. Arch Gen Psychiatry 2002;59(5):434–40.

59. Hollander E, Allen A, Kwon J, et al. Clomipramine vs desipramine crossover trial in body dysmorphic disorder: selective efficacy of a serotonin reuptake inhibitor in imagines ugliness. Arch Gen Psychiatry 1999;56(11):1033–9.

60. Rood -Y, Visser S. Principes van cognitieve gedragstherapie bij patienten met een somatoforme stoornis in de GGZ. In: Feltz-Cornelis CM, van der Horst H, editors. De Tijdstroom; 2008.

61. Felitti VJ, Jakstis K, Pepper V, et al. Obesity: problem, solution, or both? Perm J 2010;14(1):24–31.

62. Anda RF, Brown DW, Dube SR, et al. Adverse childhood experiences and chronic obstructive pulmonary diseases in adults. Am J Prev Med 2008;34: 396–403.

63. Anda RF, Brown DW, Felitti VJ, et al. Adverse childhood experiences and prescribed psychotropic

medications in adults. Am J Prev Med 2007;32(5): 389–94.

64. Anda RF, Fleisher VI, Felitti VJ, et al. Childhood abuse, household dysfunction, and indicators of impaired worker performance in adulthood. Perm J 2004;8(1):30–8.

65. Felitti VJ, Anda RF. The lifelong effects of adverse childhood experiences, Chapter 10. In: Chadwick's child maltreatment: sexual abuse and psychological maltreatment. 4th edition. Florissant (MO): STM Leaning; 2014.

66. Andrews B. Bodily shame as a mediator between abusive experiences and depression. J Abnorm Psychol 1995;104(2):277–85.

67. Weingarden H, Renshaw KD, Wilhelm S, et al. Anxiety and shame as risk factors for depression, suicidality, and functional impairment in body dysmorphic disorder and obsessive compulsive disorder. J Nerv Ment Dis 2016;204(11):832.

68. Weingarden H, Renshaw KD, Davidson E, et al. Relative relationships of general shame and body shame with body dysmorphic phenomenology and psychosocial outcomes. J Obsessive Compuls Relat Disord 2017;14:1–6.

69. Weingarden H, Shaw AM, Phillips KA, et al. Shame and defectiveness beliefs in treatment seeking patients with body dysmorphic disorder. J Nerv Ment Dis 2018;206(6):417–22.

Unhappy Patients Can Turn into Angry Patients
How to Deal with Both

Amanda E. Dilger, MD[a,b,1], Jonathan M. Sykes, MD[c,d,*]

KEYWORDS

- Facial plastic surgery • Aesthetic surgery • Outcomes • Difficult patients
- Body dysmorphic disorder

KEY POINTS

- Achieving a successful outcome in aesthetic surgery depends on numerous factors, including patient selection, procedure choice by the patient, technical performance, and postoperative patient care.
- Patient perception of results can be influenced by physician–patient interactions, starting from the patient's first communication with the practice and continuing throughout subsequent visits.
- Issues with communication in the physician–patient relationship are fairly common and often multifactorial in nature.
- Careful patient selection and maintaining an open, empathetic, and constructive physician–patient relationship are the keys to successful practice and positive outcomes.

INTRODUCTION

Patient satisfaction is the ultimate measure of success in cosmetic facial plastic surgery. Achieving a successful outcome in aesthetic surgery depends on numerous factors, including patient selection, procedure choice by the patient, technical performance by the surgeon, and postoperative patient care. Patient perception of results can be influenced by all physician–patient interactions, starting from the patient's first communication with the practice and continuing throughout the consultation, procedure, and postprocedure visits.

Most of the emphasis of surgical training focuses on diagnosis—identifying variations in physical conditions (changes in the aging face, nasal deformities, eyelid ptosis, etc), and on treatment—executing the technical aspects of surgical procedures. Although these skills are essential to a well-trained and successful facial plastic surgeon, the importance of proper patient selection, management of patient expectations, and empathetic communication throughout the preoperative and postoperative periods in cosmetic surgery are often overlooked in education and cannot be understated.

ETIOLOGY OF DIFFICULT PHYSICIAN–PATIENT RELATIONSHIPS

Issues with communication in the physician–patient relationship are fairly common and often multifactorial in nature. In the primary care setting, several studies have shown that approximately 1 in every 6 patient encounters is considered "difficult" by surveyed physicians.[1–4] Patient characteristics that have been cited as contributing factors to these challenging interactions include insistence on being prescribed unnecessary drugs, apparent dissatisfaction in care, unrealistic expectations, persistent complaints despite efforts to help, ignoring medical advice, being verbally

[a] Facial Plastic and Reconstructive Surgery, Beverly Hills, CA, USA; [b] Roseville Facial Plastic Surgery, Roseville, CA, USA; [c] Facial Plastic Surgery, UC Davis Medical Center, Sacramento, CA, USA; [d] Facial Plastic Surgery, Roxbury Institute, Beverly Hills, CA, USA
[1] Present address: 5 Medical Plaza, Suite 100, Roseville, CA 95661.
* Corresponding author. 5 Medical Plaza, Suite 100, Roseville, CA 95661.
E-mail address: jmsykes@ucdavis.edu

Facial Plast Surg Clin N Am 28 (2020) 461–468
https://doi.org/10.1016/j.fsc.2020.06.004

abusive, and being disrespectful.[5] Additionally, studies have found that patients in difficult encounters are more likely to have an underlying depressive or anxiety disorder[1,3] and somatic symptom severity of greater than 6 on a 10-point scale.[2] Patients with underlying psychiatric disorders, in particular body dysmorphic disorder (BDD), are of particular concern in cosmetic plastic surgery, because these patients are unlikely to have realistic expectations or to be satisfied with the results of surgery.

Because the physician–patient interaction is dyadic, physicians may also contribute to difficult encounters. A recent study found that physicians with more frequent difficult patient encounters had significantly higher self-reported rates of depression, stress, and anxiety; worked more hours; and were younger (age <40) than physicians who reported less frequent difficult patient encounters.[6] Additionally, poor physician attitude toward patient psychosocial issues has been found to independently increase the likelihood of difficult interaction.[2]

Specific physician-centric factors that challenge the physician–patient relationship may be difficult to further elucidate given that the majority of research is done via inherently flawed surveys and self-reporting; however, it is obvious that open, empathetic communication on the part of the physician is essential to creating a positive patient interaction. Well-established interpersonal strategies for improving relationships with difficult patients include increasing nonjudgmental listening and communicating directly.[7] A recent publication proposed the use of the ROAR approach (Reflective, Objective, Assessment, Reassurance) to the difficult patient interaction— this involves reflecting the patients distress (ie, "I am sorry; you seem frustrated"), engaging the patient in the objective evaluation, providing an assessment that includes acknowledgment of the uncertain aspects of the plan of care, and providing reassurance to emphasize that there is an open line of communication between the physician and the patient.[8] This approach offers a multitude of benefits, including helping to validate the patient's emotions, facilitating ownership over the patient's pertinent history and examination, uncovering undisclosed anxieties, and clarifying patient motivations. A compassionate and patient-centered approach to communication, such as the ROAR approach, is therefore essential to facilitating positive interactions in facial plastic surgery.

Understanding the patient's perspective is particularly important in aesthetic medicine and surgery, which involves a large amount of subjectivity in both the diagnosis and evaluation of surgical results. A patient's self-image affects their perception of appearance, what they desire to modify, and their satisfaction with any procedure. For this reason, it is crucial that the aesthetic practitioner try to understand their patient's feelings and emotions to communicate well.

The magnitude of the impaired physician–patient relationship is felt by both involved parties. Patients from difficult encounters are significantly more likely to be dissatisfied overall with the care they receive and are more critical of all aspects of the physician encounter, including technical competence, bedside manner, time spent with the clinician, and explanation of care.[2] Physicians who report greater frustration and more frequent difficult patient interactions are significantly more likely to experience symptoms of professional burnout and feel dissatisfied with their profession.[5] As such, communication skills are essential to a successful, satisfying career in cosmetic facial plastic surgery and a greater emphasis should be placed on the development of the physician–patient relationship in the literature and in medical education.

PATIENT SELECTION

The most effective way to manage unhappy and angry patients is to, as much as possible, avoid operating on patients who are likely to be dissatisfied with their surgical outcome. The decision of when not to operate is rarely discussed in surgical training and requires the use of surgeon's judgment and experience. In addition to evaluating the patient from a medical and aesthetic perspective to determine if cosmetic surgery is safe and appropriate in each particular case, the surgeon must from the earliest encounter be attuned to the psychological fitness of the patient.

In the best-seller *Blink: The Power of Thinking Without Really Thinking*, Malcolm Gladwell argues that in many instances the subcognitive perception of the trained individual is often much more valuable and accurate than an in-depth quantitative analysis.[9] As such, it is often within the first 1 to 2 minutes of the initial consultation that the surgeon can decide if the patient will be able to tolerate the emotional and psychological stress of surgery. The opinions of the physician's trusted office staff should also be taken into account. If a patient's behavior has led the office staff to feel uncomfortable (ie, condescending or rude behavior), there is a possibility that the patient is aware of these problematic characteristics and takes care to hide them during the initial encounter with the physician. These difficult personality traits have a tendency to become more apparent in the postoperative period.[10]

Before even the initial consultation, troublesome personality characteristics can manifest during telephone calls and interactions with office staff. Both in anecdotal[11] and clinical studies[12] it has been found that patients with demanding personality types (ie, requesting very specific appointment times that are difficult to satisfy, making and canceling several appointments, complaining regarding consultation costs) are at higher risk for poor outcomes. For this reason, it is important to take every interaction into account when assessing a patient's readiness for aesthetic surgery. During the consultation, the patient's appearance and behavior is important. The patient may seem to be unkempt, unhappy, hostile, or have an inappropriate affect—these are all signs of a potentially difficult patient and should be noted and documented. The surgeon should be concerned if patients have unrealistic or poorly defined expectations, have difficulty listening or attempt to dominate the conversation, or have a minimal or imagined deformity. Taken together within the context of the patient's interactions with staff members and overall health, an astute evaluation of the patient during the consultation will help the surgeon to ascertain the physical and psychological readiness of the patient for cosmetic plastic surgery.

IDENTIFYING PROBLEMATIC PERSONALITY TYPES

Examples of personality characteristics that can be difficult to manage in the cosmetic surgery patient have been previously discussed in the literature[13] and are as follows:

1. Patients with unrealistic or unfocused expectations
2. Unhappy patients
3. Patients with poor self-image
4. Overly flattering patients
5. Perfectionists
6. Rude patients
7. Very important persons (VIPs)
8. Know-it-all patients
9. BDD
10. Patients with a history of trauma

If several of these characteristics are present in the patient, it is best to either decline performing surgery or to schedule a second consultation to determine the possible impact of these personality traits on patient satisfaction with treatment.

The motivation for undergoing aesthetic surgery is an important determinate of postoperative satisfaction. A recent study of motivation and expectations in secondary rhinoplasty patients stratified groups by preoperative motive of requesting a smaller nose (ie, because of a dorsal hump) versus wanting to improve their nose because it was "not perfect enough." Patients who said that their nose was not perfect enough before surgery were significantly more likely to perceive the surgery outcome as unsuccessful than those who desired a smaller nose.[14] It is therefore essential that the surgeon pay close attention to the patient's expectations, including taking into account photographs of goals that the patient is hoping to achieve. Similar to the patient with unrealistic expectations, perfectionists may also be unable to accept minor asymmetries or slight imperfections that are well within the range of expected postoperative results. It is the role of the surgeon to communicate the limitations of aesthetic surgery with the patient and to ensure that these limitations are understood before proceeding with any procedure.

Patients who are not diagnosed with an overt mood disorder but have an overall unhappy demeanor may have a tendency to focus on the negative aspects of subjective situations. Because the outcomes of aesthetic surgery are subjective, undergoing a cosmetic procedure presents an opportunity for dissatisfaction and negativity. The surgeon must use instinct to assess a patient's demeanor during the preoperative consultation.[10] Similarly, patients with a poor overall self-image are less likely to perceive significant benefit from aesthetic surgery. This characteristic may manifest as an unkept or disheveled appearance, which can also be a clue to an undisclosed psychiatric condition.[11]

Overly flattering patients—those who excessively praise the surgeon's knowledge, abilities, and reputation—present a tempting situation for the surgeon. However, these patients are often quick to change opinions in the event of an unsatisfactory outcome. On careful history taking, the surgeon asks if the patient has visited many surgeons to be "treated by only the best," despite having no significant experience or knowledge of the surgeon's technical skills or outcomes. These patients may make demeaning or derogatory comments toward other surgeons that they have previously seen. Although there are no specific studies dedicated to this patient characteristic, anecdotal evidence in the literature suggests that, if these patients are unhappy with the outcome of surgery, their excessive flattery can be replaced with rage and anger.[11]

VIP patients (ie, those who are highly visible to the public including actors, politicians, musicians) may be more likely to require extra attention in the preoperative and postoperative period. Additional requests, including avoidance of preoperative laboratory testing, early splint removal, exemption from postoperative restrictions, and dedicated nursing care, are also commonly made by these patients. Although appropriate courtesies should be made, it is important to avoid the pressure to cut corners, because these changes in protocol can be detrimental to the patient's outcome.[11] It is best to avoid working with VIP (and pseudo-VIP patients) unless the surgeon and office staff are able to provide the extra level of attentiveness that is required.[15]

BODY DYSMORPHIC DISORDER IN PLASTIC SURGERY PATIENTS

It is essential that plastic surgeons are able to recognize the characteristics of BDD, because these patients characteristically are unlikely to benefit from a surgical procedure and should be referred for appropriate psychological therapy. The latest version of the *Diagnostic and Statistical Manual of Mental Health Disorders* (DSM) placed BDD in a new category of obsessive–compulsive and related disorders, and diagnosis requires performance of repetitive behavior and/or thoughts, including "mirror checking, excessive grooming, skin picking, [and] reassurance seeking." These patients are also prone to avoiding social situations owing to concerns regarding their appearance or use a variety of techniques to camouflage their perceived flaws.[16] Presentations can vary widely, from mild fixation on a particular feature to obsession with transforming all aspects of the appearance. The point prevalence of BDD on the basis of DSM-III, DSM-IV, or DSM-5 criteria range from 0.7% to 2.9%[17–20] in the general population and 2.5% to 5.3% in college students.[21–23] In patients seeking cosmetic plastic surgery, the prevalence is likely to be significantly higher, although the exact incidence is still unknown.[24,25] One study of 226 patients seeking rhinoplasty for aesthetic and/or functional reasons found that one-third of the patients met criteria for moderate BDD based on the Yale–Brown Obsessive Compulsive scale modified for BDD.[26]

As noted, BDD can have a significant negative impact on the physician–patient relationship and the perceived outcome of cosmetic procedures. In the aforementioned group of patients seeking cosmetic rhinoplasty, it was found that preoperative BDD symptom scores inversely correlated with patients' quality of life and satisfaction after surgery.[27] This finding is consistent with prior studies, which showed that nonpsychiatric treatment of BDD is not effective—most patients exhibit unchanged or worsened symptom severity after undergoing cosmetic procedures.[28,29] Although some patients with BDD may initially declare satisfaction with the surgery, these patients still exhibit high psychiatric handicap and BDD symptomatology at 5-year follow-up.[30] As such, it is important to remember that BDD is in fact a contraindication for aesthetic surgery that warrants psychiatric intervention despite the inclination that the surgeon may be able to make a positive objective change with surgery.

HISTORY OF TRAUMA

The effects of trauma, particularly childhood abuse or neglect, on body image,[31,32] body shame,[33–36] and development[37] are complex and beyond the scope of this discussion. However, given the significant impact of the patient's self-image and motivation on the outcome of cosmetic surgery, it is worth considering screening for a history of trauma as part of the preoperative psychological assessment. A recent study of 100 patients undergoing secondary rhinoplasty sought to better understand the motivation of patients with straight, functional noses. When compared with patients with dorsal humps, patients with normal noses were 3.8 more likely to have a history of confirmed trauma, abuse, or neglect.[12] Trauma was also inversely related to surgical success, with the odds of a successful surgical outcome 3.6 times higher in patients without a history of abuse or neglect.[14] This relationship held true even when controlling for variations in preoperative nasal shape (ie, presence of dorsal hump vs straight) and number of prior surgeries. In this study as well as in 1 small prior study, there was a significant correlation between those with confirmed trauma histories and those who met the criteria for BDD.[38] As such, a history of trauma likely does not represent a distinct contraindication to cosmetic plastic surgery, but rather a clue to shed light on the etiology of maladaptive or nonfunctional personality traits that may make a patient a poor surgical candidate.

MANAGING DIFFICULT PATIENTS

If concerns regarding a patient's ability to psychologically tolerate aesthetic surgery are raised during the initial preoperative consultation, the first option for management is to schedule a second consultation. This strategy allows both the patient and the surgeon to reevaluate the situation and address lingering questions or concerns from the initial encounter. If the surgeon's concerns are alleviated by the second consultation, then surgery can be scheduled with greater confidence that the outcome will be satisfactory to the patient. However, if the patient continues to exhibit difficult or dangerous personality characteristics, then the second consultation was of great value in that it provided additional evidence to support the decision to avoid surgery in a potentially problematic patient.

Another option for patients who may be unable to tolerate surgery is to offer minimally invasive, reversible in-office procedures such as injectable facial fillers and/or Botox (botulinum toxin; Allergan, Inc.; Irvine, CA). In addition to providing temporary treatment for a variety of aesthetic issues, injectables or other minimally invasive procedures allow the surgeon to gauge the patient's ability to withstand procedures and judge treatment results. Patients who are able to perceive positive results may be more likely to respond well to more invasive surgical procedures.[10]

REFUSING SURGERY TO POTENTIAL PATIENTS

Aesthetic surgery is, in almost all instances, elective; therefore, if a patient is not a suitable candidate for medical reasons or psychological reasons, the surgeon is tasked with refusing surgery to the potential patient. This issue can be sensitive, because the surgeon may be confident that a procedure will objectively improve the patient's appearance. There may also be financial factors that motivate the surgeon to recruit potential patients. Additionally, the patient who is seeking aesthetic surgery is likely to be disappointed or angry with the outcome of the consultation if surgery is not recommended. It is important that, in the case of refusing surgery to a patient, the surgeon is open about their concerns and provides referrals to other potential surgeons. An approach that may help to diffuse the situation is to place the onus on the surgeon by saying, for example, "I am concerned about my ability to achieve your desired result." This strategy directs the blame away from the patient's difficult personality characteristics and toward the surgeon. Although these conversations can be difficult, it is far easier to dissuade a difficult patient from surgery than it is to manage patient dissatisfaction and anger in the postoperative setting.[39]

MANAGING PATIENT DISSATISFACTION

Cases of patient dissatisfaction in aesthetic surgery can be devastating to both the patient and the surgeon. These instances represent a minority of the surgeon's practice; however, they can occupy a significant amount of clinical time, energy, and thoughts. Communication is essential in the management of dissatisfaction in the postoperative cosmetic surgery patient, and the key to effective communication is listening. There are several techniques for optimizing listening skills to maximize the value of the physician–patient relationship. Listening with curiosity and genuine interest will help the surgeon to better understand the etiology of the patient's concerns. It is also important to give the patient adequate time and space to express their concerns freely, and listening in silence provides this opportunity.[40] Reflective listening, which involves paraphrasing what the patient says back to them, can help the patient to understand that the surgeon is listening and understanding their points. Phrases such as "if I could summarize what I am hearing" or "it sounds like you are saying" followed by "is this correct?" or "have I properly characterized your complaints?" can be helpful in these conversations.[13]

In some cases, it may be useful to use, with permission from the patient, communication with the patient's family and/or friends as a method to better alleviate a difficult situation. The patient's support system may be able to provide insight and context into the scenario that was otherwise unavailable and offer an additional objective opinion on the surgical outcome.[39]

Thorough and accurate documentation of all patient interactions, including e-mails and phone calls, as well as photodocumentation before and after the procedure is essential for multiple reasons. These records can be used to objectively demonstrate improvements in the preoperative appearance that the patient may have difficulty recognizing. Additionally, in cases of malpractice claims against plastic surgeons, studies suggest that the quality of informed consent and medical documentation can weigh heavily on the judicial decision.[41,42]

ANGRY PATIENTS

Patients who are unhappy or unsatisfied with their aesthetic surgery outcome can occasionally become angry with their treatment team. This anger can be a function of an underlying psychopathology that becomes exacerbated in the postoperative period. In patients with BDD, for example, the severity of the BDD correlates significantly with levels of anger and hostility.[43] As with any dissatisfied patient, it is important to allow the patient to express their concerns and feel heard by the surgeon. Maintaining a high level of empathy and compassion will provide an opportunity to salvage the physician–patient relationship, despite increasing levels of tension, and hopefully prevent further escalation of the situation.

In very rare cases, patients can become hostile and even threatening with their plastic surgery team. Although these cases are infrequent, it is important that the surgeon use instincts and experience to assess which patients could pose a legitimate safety threat. In the event that a patient becomes threatening, it is important to immediately inform office staff of the threat and show them pictures of the patient, so they can be on high alert for suspicious or unusual behavior. Other suggestions include changing the locks to the office or hiring security during scheduled visits with the patient.[11] As with other unhappy or dissatisfied patients, it is important to have an open manner of communication with angry patients—allow them to ventilate their frustrations, address their concerns honestly, and provide referrals to other reputable plastic surgeons for additional opinions. Although it may be difficult and uncomfortable to interact with these patients in a follow-up appointment, these visits provide a valuable opportunity to attain some level of closure, even if that means terminating the relationship with the patient. Additionally, frequent postoperative visits provide an opportunity to review standardized preoperative and postoperative photography to better quantify the improvements that the patient has been unable to comprehend.

Although in the case of a particularly confrontational or unpleasant patient, it may seem tempting to "counterattack," it is of utmost importance to resist this temptation. Engaging in a confrontation with an upset or angry patient is counterproductive and will often provoke further distrust and aggression from the patient.

MALPRACTICE LITIGATION CASES

It is important to understand the factors influencing litigation and judiciary decisions given the nature of medical malpractice litigation in today's environment. When patient dissatisfaction persists, it is appropriate to consult risk management and the physician's liability insurance carrier to ensure legal protection in the event of malpractice litigation. To be liable for malpractice, the surgeon must fail to meet the community standard of care and produce direct injurious results. Additionally, surgeons may be held accountable for "breach of warranty" if the results produced are not akin to those that were guaranteed preoperatively.[44]

Although there are no data in the literature to support this notion, it is very likely that poor communication and misunderstanding of

expectations plays a significant role in malpractice litigation in cosmetic plastic surgery. In the largest study to date of rhytidectomy malpractice cases, 69% of cases cited "intraoperative negligence" as the cause for allegation.[45] This complaint is nonspecific and does not reflect a particular outcome or injury—for example, facial nerve injury is listed as a separate allegation and was present in only 11% of these cases. As such, it is plausible that this complaint represents general dissatisfaction with the outcome and care provided.[46] Given the known detriment of unmet expectations on patient satisfaction, it is of utmost importance to communicate openly.

DISCUSSION

Difficult physician–patient relationships are common and multifactorial, with contributing factors from both the physician and the patient. It is essential for the facial plastic surgeon to develop the communication skills necessary to evaluate each patient on an individual basis to assess for personality characteristics that may be difficult to manage in the postoperative setting. Careful patient selection and maintaining an open, empathetic and constructive physician–patient relationship are the keys to successful practice and positive outcomes.

DISCLOSURE

The authors have nothing to disclose.

REFERENCES

1. Hahn SR, Kroenke K, Spitzer RL, et al. The difficult patient: prevalence, psychopathology, and functional impairment. J Gen Intern Med 1996;11(1):1–8.
2. Jackson JL, Kroenke K. Difficult patient encounters in the ambulatory clinic: clinical predictors and outcomes. Arch Intern Med 1999;159(10):1069–75.
3. Crutcher JE, Bass MJ. The difficult patient and the troubled physician. J Fam Pract 1980;11(6):933–8.
4. Jackson JL, Kroenke K. The effect of unmet expectations among adults presenting with physical symptoms. Ann Intern Med 2001;134(9 Pt 2):889–97.
5. An PG, Rabatin JS, Manwell LB, et al. Burden of difficult encounters in primary care: data from the minimizing error, maximizing outcomes study. Arch Intern Med 2009;169(4):410–4.
6. Krebs EE, Garrett JM, Konrad TR. The difficult doctor? Characteristics of physicians who report frustration with patients: an analysis of survey data. BMC Health Serv Res 2006;6:128.
7. Adams J, Murray R 3rd. The general approach to the difficult patient. Emerg Med Clin North Am 1998;16(4):689–700, v.

8. McCarthy JG, Cheatham JG, Singla M. How to approach difficult patient encounters: ROAR. Gastroenterology 2018;155(2):258–61.

9. Gladwell M. Blink: the power of thinking without really thinking. New York: Little, Brown, and Company; 2005.

10. Sykes JM. Managing the psychological aspects of plastic surgery patients. Curr Opin Otolaryngol Head Neck Surg 2009;17(4):321–5.

11. Connell BF, Gunter J, Mayer T, et al. Roundtable: discussion of "the difficult patient. Facial Plast Surg Clin North Am 2008;16(2):249–58, viii.

12. Constantian MB, Lin CP. Why some patients are unhappy: part 1. Relationship of preoperative nasal deformity to number of operations and a history of abuse or neglect. Plast Reconstr Surg 2014; 134(4):823–35.

13. Sykes J, Javidnia H, A contemporary review of the management of the difficult patient. JAMA Facial Plast Surg 2013;15(2):81–4.

14. Constantian MB, Lin CP. Why some patients are unhappy: part 2. Relationship of nasal shape and trauma history to surgical success. Plast Reconstr Surg 2014;134(4):836–51.

15. Goode RL. The unhappy patient following facial plastic surgery: what to do? Facial Plast Surg Clin North Am 2008;16(2):183–6, vi.

16. Association AP. Diagnostic and statistical manual of mental disorders. 5th edition. Arlington (VA): American Psychiatric Publishing; 2013.

17. Schieber K, Kollei I, de Zwaan M, et al. Classification of body dysmorphic disorder - what is the advantage of the new DSM-5 criteria? J Psychosom Res 2015;78(3):223–7.

18. Brohede S, Wingren G, Wijma B, et al. Prevalence of body dysmorphic disorder among Swedish women: a population-based study. Compr Psychiatry 2015; 58.108–15.

19. Buhlmann U, Glaesmer H, Mewes R, et al. Updates on the prevalence of body dysmorphic disorder: a population-based survey. Psychiatry Res 2010; 178(1):171–5.

20. Faravelli C, Salvatori S, Galassi F, et al. Epidemiology of somatoform disorders: a community survey in Florence. Soc Psychiatry Psychiatr Epidemiol 1997;32(1):24–9.

21. Bohne A, Wilhelm S, Keuthen NJ, et al. Prevalence of body dysmorphic disorder in a German college student sample. Psychiatry Res 2002;109(1):101–4.

22. Cansever A, Uzun O, Donmez E, et al. The prevalence and clinical features of body dysmorphic disorder in college students: a study in a Turkish sample. Compr Psychiatry 2003;44(1):60–4.

23. Sarwer DB, Cash TF, Magee L, et al. Female college students and cosmetic surgery: an investigation of experiences, attitudes, and body image. Plast Reconstr Surg 2005;115(3):931–8.

24. Ishigooka J, Iwao M, Suzuki M, et al. Demographic features of patients seeking cosmetic surgery. Psychiatry Clin Neurosci 1998;52(3):283–7.

25. Veale D, De Haro L, Lambrou C. Cosmetic rhinoplasty in body dysmorphic disorder. Br J Plast Surg 2003;56(6):546–51.

26. Picavet VA, Prokopakis EP, Gabriels L, et al. High prevalence of body dysmorphic disorder symptoms in patients seeking rhinoplasty. Plast Reconstr Surg 2011;128(2):509–17.

27. Picavet VA, Gabriels L, Grietens J, et al. Preoperative symptoms of body dysmorphic disorder determine postoperative satisfaction and quality of life in aesthetic rhinoplasty. Plast Reconstr Surg 2013; 131(4):861–8.

28. Crerand CE, Phillips KA, Menard W, et al. Nonpsychiatric medical treatment of body dysmorphic disorder. Psychosomatics 2005;46(6):549–55.

29. Phillips KA, Grant J, Siniscalchi J, et al. Surgical and nonpsychiatric medical treatment of patients with body dysmorphic disorder. Psychosomatics 2001; 42(6):504–10.

30. Tignol J, Biraben-Gotzamanis L, Martin-Guehl C, et al. Body dysmorphic disorder and cosmetic surgery: evolution of 24 subjects with a minimal defect in appearance 5 years after their request for cosmetic surgery. Eur Psychiatry 2007;22(8): 520–4.

31. Wenninger K, Heiman JR. Relating body image to psychological and sexual functioning in child sexual abuse survivors. J Trauma Stress 1998;11(3): 543–62.

32. Dyer A, Borgmann E, Kleindienst N, et al. Body image in patients with posttraumatic stress disorder after childhood sexual abuse and co-occurring eating disorder. Psychopathology 2013;46(3):186–91.

33. Franzoni E, Gualandi S, Caretti V, et al. The relationship between alexithymia, shame, trauma, and body image disorders: investigation over a large clinical sample. Neuropsychiatr Dis Treat 2013;9:185–93.

34. Dorahy MJ. The impact of dissociation, shame, and guilt on interpersonal relationships in chronically traumatized individuals: a pilot study. J Trauma Stress 2010;23(5):653–6.

35. Andrews B. Bodily shame as a mediator between abusive experiences and depression. J Abnorm Psychol 1995;104(2):277–85.

36. Constantian M. Childhood abuse, body shame and addictive plastic surgery. New York: Routledge; 2019.

37. Kaplow JB, Saxe GN, Putnam FW, et al. The longterm consequences of early childhood trauma: a case study and discussion. Psychiatry 2006;69(4): 362–75.

38. Didie ER, Tortolani CC, Pope CG, et al. Childhood abuse and neglect in body dysmorphic disorder. Child Abuse Negl 2006;30(10):1105–15.

39. Sykes JM. Patient selection in facial plastic surgery. Facial Plast Surg Clin North Am 2008;16(2):173–6, v.

40. Buffington A, Wenner P, Brandenburg D, et al. The Art of Listening. Minn Med 2016;99(6):46–8.

41. Reisch LM, Carney PA, Oster NV, et al. Medical malpractice concerns and defensive medicine: a nationwide survey of breast pathologists. Am J Clin Pathol 2015;144(6):916–22.

42. Vila-Nova da Silva DB, Nahas FX, Ferreira LM. Factors influencing judicial decisions on medical disputes in plastic surgery. Aesthet Surg J 2015; 35(4):477–83.

43. Phillips KA, Siniscalchi JM, McElroy SL. Depression, anxiety, anger, and somatic symptoms in patients with body dysmorphic disorder. Psychiatr Q 2004; 75(4):309–20.

44. Gorney M. Claims prevention for the aesthetic surgeon: preparing for the less-than-perfect outcome. Facial Plast Surg 2002;18(2):135–42.

45. Kandinov A, Mutchnick S, Nangia V, et al. Analysis of Factors Associated With Rhytidectomy Malpractice Litigation Cases. JAMA Facial Plast Surg 2017; 19(4):255–9.

46. Sykes JM. Is studying rhytidectomy malpractice cases enough to understand why patients are dissatisfied? More patient communication, less malpractice litigation. JAMA Facial Plast Surg 2017;19(4):259–60.

The Art of Teaching, Training, and Putting the Scalpel in Residents' Hands

Sherard Austin Tatum III, MD, FAAP, FACS

KEYWORDS

- Facial plastic and reconstructive surgery • Plastic and reconstructive surgery • Surgical training
- Teaching • Surgical education • Surgical residency

KEY POINTS

- Surgical training is under tremendous pressure due to ever-increasing medical knowledge and demands on the time of trainees. They must continually learn more in less time.
- Surgical training must become more efficient. The preparation for each case has to be maximal. Preoperative, intraoperative, and postoperative discussion improves the educational benefit of the trainee experience.
- For the teaching surgeon, putting the scalpel in residents' hands requires knowledge, judgment, and a leap of faith in the resident. Even under the closest supervision, the teacher depends on the caution and prudence of the student.
- There is an unprecedented array of education and training opportunities for the resident to prepare for being handed the scalpel. Such opportunities include traditional reading sources, procedural videos, animal and cadaver dissection, live and virtual simulation, and so forth.

INTRODUCTION

There is no getting around it. Handing over the scalpel to a trainee requires intestinal fortitude, patience, and trust. It also requires preparation by the learner and the teacher and the teachers' confidence in their own abilities. A learner who is unprepared for a case is not a good candidate for being handed a scalpel. A surgeon who is rushed or uncomfortable with a case is likely to be a less patient, comfortable, and effective teacher, let alone knowing the trainee's capabilities. The teaching surgeon is ultimately responsible for the outcome, and there is a lot that can be done to increase the chances of a good surgical and educational outcome.

HISTORICAL PERSPECTIVE

See one, do one, teach one: was that not the mantra of bygone training? In reality, surgeons are the beneficiaries of generous, patient and dedicated teaching surgeons and their patients.[1] Most of surgeons have stories of crazy behavior and abusiveness from characters of the past, but even these colorful personalities by and large were committed teachers. They often employed Socratic methods that were not always pleasant. Trainees learned on the fly without work hour limitations, smartphones, or electronic medical records. Learners read before cases, or if they did not, they heard about it. When teachers handed teachers the knife, they had no idea if (s)he knew

Department of Otolaryngology, Cleft and Craniofacial Center, Division of Facial Plastic and Reconstructive Surgery, Upstate Medical University, State University of New York, 750 East Adams Street, CWB, Syracuse, NY 13210, USA
E-mail address: tatums@upstate.edu
Twitter: @SherardTatum (S.A.T.)

Facial Plast Surg Clin N Am 28 (2020) 469–475
https://doi.org/10.1016/j.fsc.2020.06.005
1064-7406/20/© 2020 Elsevier Inc. All rights reserved.

how to use it. But residents learned gradually by a slow, progressive increase in responsibility. As the teaching surgeons got to know residents and their skill level better, they became more comfortable with letting trainees do more. A series of cases with the same attending was a mini-apprenticeship.

Residents did a year or 2 of general surgery where, if they did what they were told (read for the case, gather the preoperative laboratory test results and imaging, and do the paperwork), they learned to cut, sew, and tie knots. They also learned how to recognize and take care of sick patients. The core competencies were knowledge, judgment, dexterity, and compassion. They advanced by a gradual increase in responsibility.[2] The history of this approach dates back to ancient times of Socrates and Hippocrates. Modern bedside teaching was championed by Osler and Halsted.

CHALLENGES

But times are changing. The public gradually has become aware of this on-the-job-training method and rebelled a little: "I don't want to be practiced on." "You're doing the surgery, not a resident, right?" Those surgeons spending a long time building a community reputation (for example, in a cosmetic surgery practice) can be particularly pressured by patient demands: "I'm paying for you, Doc. I expect you to do my surgery." For better or worse, the Internet provides and empowers patients with a tremendous amount of information about medical conditions and care providers. Practice profiles include information about participation in resident education. This can steer patients away from academic practices.

There also is ever-increasing pressure to be more productive to compensate for diminishing reimbursements, the drag of electronic medical records, and inefficiencies of regulation and defensive practice.[2] The drive for high-quality outcomes, low complication rates, and low length of stay statistics all pressure teaching surgeons toward operating more and teaching less.[3] Teaching takes time, a luxury few have in abundance. Additionally, not everyone is a great teacher. Few have formal training in how to teach. Some are naturally gifted teachers, but most learn by observing and trying to emulate those seen as good teachers—more see one, do one, teach one.[4] There is training available in how to teach surgical residents through the American College of Surgeons and the Association of American Medical Colleges, among others organizations.

Surgical knowledge and technology are expanding rapidly. Trainees have many more procedures to learn during their training, which means fewer opportunities with each procedure. Work hour restrictions have reduced the time spent in training. Residents have to spend more time with electronic medical records than with their patients. The trends toward endoscopic, minimally invasive, and robotic surgery have made it harder for a learner to participate in cases, with ever-steepening learning curves. The consequence is that current trainees are having to learn more with less time.[5] That leaves several choices: do not learn enough, learn longer, and learn more efficiently. It does not seem that there is an appetite for less well-trained surgeons or significantly lengthened training, although the popularity of fellowship training probably is due at least in part to this volume-time squeeze.[6]

The question becomes, How can the teaching benefit of allowing a resident to operate be safely and efficiently maximize? For a brief digression, recall past and ongoing efforts to assess dexterity in resident applicants. There have been numerous attempts to select the more dexterous applicants in a pool for residency training with the presumption that they will make better surgeons. Clearly the thinking is that starting with better dexterity results in a more dexterous final product. The training process might be a little easier on the teachers as well. These assessment attempts, however, have yielded equivocal results. They are not used widely, but similar efforts are being made to assess success in training with milestones—more on that later. More broadly, efforts are being made to enhance resident selection in general, including structured interviews, personality inventories, and situational judgment tests.[7]

OPPORTUNITIES AND STRATEGIES

Teaching must be more efficient. The learning benefit needs to be maximized for each case. Preoperative preparation has to be emphasized. Learners must demonstrate that they know the basic science facts pertinent to a procedure. Reading, attending lectures or small group discussions, watching videos, and employing virtual and real simulations are extremely important preparations for getting the most from a procedure whether watching or performing. One of the most important preparations for a case is assisting and seeing the procedure done well by an experienced surgeon either in the operating room (OR) or on video. Engagement from those holding retractors and observing must be insisted on. Allowing daydreaming when important technical lessons are being demonstrated cannot be afforded. If feasible, important bilateral cases should be shared between 2 residents to maximize exposure. It is an even better learning experience if a more experienced trainee can take a less experienced trainee through a procedure. Having to think through the procedure enough to explain it deepens the understanding of the procedure (back to see one, do one, teach one).

Preoperative discussion between the attending and resident surgeons can be hugely beneficial. Although the "preoperation huddle" (think extended time out) has been proposed as a quality improvement measure, it also is a learning opportunity for the resident. The preparation of the OR and patient, operative plan, and maneuvers to avoid complications all are worthy components of the huddle. Learners demonstrate that they know how a procedure is done even if they have not yet done it. Preoperative visualization of how the operative note will be written can be a useful exercise as well. Intraoperative preparation for allowing a resident to operate occurs when that resident is assisting/observing. Discussions during the procedure of what is being done and why and what pitfalls to avoid can be very useful as are what-if scenarios to broaden the scope and educational benefit of a given clinical situation.

Another quality improvement initiative is the immediate postoperative debriefing where structured feedback and the discussion of successes and opportunities for improvement can help retention of lessons learned from the case. This is an opportunity for coaching of the learner. Particularly helpful references related to a case can be shared with the trainee at this point, if not already done. Dictating the operative note and returning to simulation and the literature after the case can help to cement the lessons learned during the case. Mistakes made during the case can be reworked in the cadaver or microscope laboratory or other simulation and improved for the next time. Reviewing and editing the operative note with the trainee affords another opportunity for reflection, reinforcement, and correction.[8]

How is it known when a resident is ready to operate? If a learner has previously scrubbed and assisted, then there might be some indication of readiness. There might be reports from other rotations and other attendings, or more senior residents can be asked about the skill level of a new resident about to be worked with, but those assessments often are limited. It is particularly difficult in doing in a unique type of case that others in the program do not do. The residents can be asked directly if they have read on the case, quizzed to verify, and asked if they have seen the

case (on YouTube, for example) or even done parts before. Despite all this intel gathering, it is still a leap of faith to put a scalpel in the resident's hand, and the residents' judgment about their own limitations, how careful (slow) to be, and when to stop or ask for help is depended on. Very close supervision typically ensues until there is a feel for the resident's skill and judgment levels. Technology can provide some aid with developing and assessing rudimentary skills. A curriculum involving assigned reading, videos, lectures, and time with simulation prior to OR time can provide reasonable preparation.[9,10] Milestone or competency testing then can provide some indication of achievement of desired skills. Preset criteria must be met before advancement to the next stage of training or the next procedure.

Unfortunately, skill level is not synonymous with experience level. Teachers have all I have had junior residents with natural dexterity who are more skillful than their seniors. Trainers also have had senior residents who struggle with dexterity and speed. Surgical judgment factors in when the dexterous resident goes a little too fast and gets into trouble, or the less dexterous resident compensates by going slower. If the amount of time is limited, when residents are allowed to operate, then the slower residents get less practice rather than what they need, which is more time. More time with videos and simulation is one answer. Whether is it cadaver or animal laboratory, smart mannequins, robot practice, or virtual reality simulation, all of these provide the added procedural experience needed by some to reach training milestones.[11] It is hoped that all trainees develop appropriate dexterity and judgment by the end of their training, but they will develop their skills at different rates. Simulation can help level this playing field.[12] Another related question is, When is the resident allowed to operate with less supervision; attending in the room but not scrubbed or attending down the hall or at home (if ever)? This is part of the progressive increase in responsibility that is surgical training. Resident performance on milestone evaluations can add to the gestalt on which teaching physicians base these decisions.[13]

Boot camps with simulation have become popular in recent years. In this scenario, early residents are put through an intensive core curriculum training experience either at the home institution or a regional host institution or third-party educational organization. These activities are designed to quickly and efficiently bring a cohort of inexperienced trainees up to a minimum threshold knowledge level to prepare them for their early duties in residency.[14] Topics like emergency airway management,[15] hemorrhage, and trauma assessment typically are covered, although any subject with a core of critical knowledge that lends itself to straightforward didactics can be taught this way. For example, there are numerous microsurgery courses available providing basic skill set training.

Another area of training worth mentioning is the overseas experience, whether a mission trip or international rotation.[16–18] These seem to become more popular every year. Senior residents and fellows typically are the ones allowed to take advantage of these opportunities. Although this type of activity is a wonderful way not only to gain surgical experience but also to acquire cultural sensitivity, it must be remembered that the supervision criteria are no different away from home versus at home. Additionally, procedures outside of training and experience should not be performed.[19] There are ethical guidelines for conducting overseas missions put forth by several oversight organizations, such as the World Health Organization and the American College of Surgeons, that are useful for mission leaders.

ADULT EDUCATION

A paradigm shift in adult education has occurred over the past 30 years. It has been discovered that young adult learners prefer to not be publicly embarrassed by being asked questions or criticized in their learning environment (I am pretty sure older generations did not like it either.) A safe, nonthreatening environment is desired for learning and feedback. They prefer small group discussions to lectures. They prefer practical learning over theory. Courses emphasizing a high teacher-to-learner ratio and hands-on components are popular. E-learning is preferred over traditional approaches.[20] There is a diminution in the importance of recall of facts with a concomitant focus on knowing where to find the facts and on team problem solving.

Adult learners want to know why they need to know something. They are self-directed and more motivated to learn practical information that serves their goals. Needs assessments are useful in determining what should be taught and placing teacher and student on the same page. Effective education involves affecting the domains of knowledge, skills, and attitudes. A successful learner acquires new knowledge, masters new psychomotor skills, and obtains new attitudes toward using the knowledge and skills. Miller's[21] pyramid (**Fig. 1**) describes the progressive increase in responsibility in educational terms. The learner begins with basic sciences (medical school and residency didactics), progressing to clinical application of

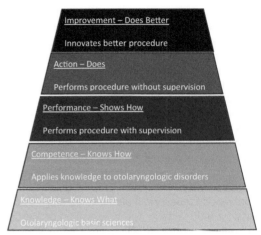

Fig. 1. Modified Miller's pyramid.[21]

basic sciences and then on to procedural training with gradual reduction in supervision. This process tends not to be linear and different phases can occur simultaneously. The Kolb[22] cycle (**Fig. 2**) describes the looping that occurs as the learner observes a procedure: reads, watches video, and works with simulation related to the procedure; performs the procedure (or parts thereof) with close supervision; does more reading, video watching, or simulation work; and performs the procedure better with tacit supervision, ultimately functioning independently and even improving the procedure.

EDUCATIONAL TECHNOLOGY

Allowing a resident to operate is providing experiential learning with some risk. This hands-on training is part of a curriculum that includes reading, lectures, videos, and the low-risk experiential learning of simulation.[23] This is a period of unprecedented advancements in education. Technology and ingenuity have provided excellent new tools for training young surgeons.[24] Animal and cadaver laboratories have been around a while, but new uses and tissue preservation procedures have enhanced utilization of these methods.[25] Even 3-dimensional (3-D) sculpting provides a low-tech form of simulation to aid trainees.[26] New artificial materials, such as model synthetic vessel tubules for practicing microanastomoses reduce the need for live animal models. Computer-aided virtual surgical planning and 3-D printed models allow a case to be planned in great detail with specific patient anatomy in the planners' hands.[27,28] It is important for the teaching surgeon to find the time to do the planning sessions with the learners.

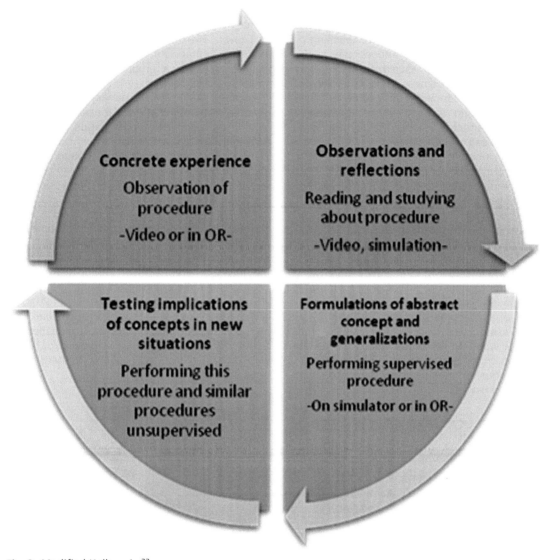

Fig. 2. Modified Kolb cycle.[22]

Live, virtual, and augmented reality simulations now provide minimal-risk practice opportunities for many procedures and scenarios.[29] Virtual reality simulation offers the opportunity to work with 3-D images of anatomy, allowing great detail for study and manipulation.[30] Procedures can be repeatedly performed virtually until a desired level of psychomotor skill is obtained.[31] As with live surgery, proper preparation, supervision, and debriefing are important parts of maximizing the simulation experience.[32] Once maximum benefit is obtained from virtual reality simulation, live simulation can be performed with smart high-fidelity mannequins, cadavers, or animals. Augmented reality glasses, for example, can overlay imaging on the surgical field to assist with

anatomy and pathology identification.[33] This simulation technology then can be used for milestone testing to assess readiness to operate (discussed later). Many institutions have built simulation laboratories on their premises. There also are mobile laboratories that can be arranged to visit a center. This visit can be coordinated with other departments to improve efficiency of utilization.

SUPERVISION

Technology also helps with intraoperative visualization. High-definition fixed overhead or head light cameras allow a bird's eye or surgeon's view to be shown on a monitor in the OR or distantly. Endoscopes continue to become smaller and offer ever-improving images. Even procedures traditionally not done with endoscopes can be visualized better for teaching or supervision with the aid of endoscopes in the field. This intraoperative visualization is a 2-way street. Not only can trainees get a better view of the attending performing a procedure but also they can perform the procedures themselves with far better attending visualization, supervision, and assessment.

Another area that has seen advances from research is assessment of technical skills.[34] There are numerous instruments designed for assessment of operative abilities and their progression.[35] The same simulation and virtual reality tools used for training can be used for trainee assessment.[36] Milestone or competency testing allows for assessment of simulation competency (agreed-on criteria the learner must achieve before being handed the scalpel) in individual procedures.[37] Video observation and rating of resident performance of procedures also can be useful. This type of assessment requires significant commitments of time and resources on the part of the institution and individual faculty, but the promise is higher-quality, more efficient education with less patient risk.[38]

SURGICAL EDUCATION/SIMULATION WEB SITES

> https://www.facs.org/education/division-of-education/publications/rise
> https://ossovr.com/aocmf3.aofoundation.org
> https://www.aafprs-learn.org/Default.aspx
> https://www.youtube.com/
> https://cleftsim.org
> https://www.voxel-man.com/simulators/ent/
> https://mededlabs.com/
> http://www.mobilesti.com/mobile-bioskills-labs/
> https://blog.capterra.com/the-top-free-surgery-simulators-for-medical-professionals/
> https://surgicaleducation.com/
> https://caehealthcare.com/surgical-simulation/
> https://www.healthysimulation.com/surgical-simulation/

SUMMARY

Handing over control of the scalpel is difficult enough on its own. Knowing when and how much to trust a trainee's skill set is even harder. Resident candidate selection tools might provide some clue as to a new trainee's skills, but gathering information from the grape vine and close personal observation are still primary methods for gaging an early trainee's skill level. Milestone testing offers promise in indicating a trainee's readiness to operate as well as signaling a program when a resident might be falling behind.

Because of the ever-expanding number and complexity of procedures and the competing regulatory and administrative demands on training time, teaching more efficiently must be learned. This requires more effort and engagement on the parts of both teacher and trainee in deriving maximal educational benefit from each operative experience. Preoperative preparation, including reading, videos, webinars, and simulation, when available, is key to gaining as much as possible from the operative experience. Teachers almost must be engaged and demand the same from the learners. Preoperative, intraoperative, and postoperative discussions between the teaching surgeon and learner are extremely valuable. Awareness of learner-preferred teaching methods and new teaching technology, patience, trust, and a desire to impart surgical excellence will serve the teaching surgeons, trainees, and patients well.

DISCLOSURE

The author has nothing to disclose.

REFERENCES

1. Kotsis SV, Chung KC. Application of the "see one, do one, teach one" concept in surgical training [Review]. Plast Reconstr Surg 2013;131(5):1194–201.
2. Weber RA, Aretz HT. Climbing the ladder from novice to expert plastic surgeon [Review]. Plast Reconstr Surg 2012;130(1):241–7.
3. Luce EA. The future of plastic surgery resident education [Review]. Plast Reconstr Surg 2016;137(3):1063–70.
4. Tsai Do BS. Reflections on the changing platform of education for the budding otolaryngologist [Review]. Otolaryngol Head Neck Surg 2015;153(5):706–7.
5. Khansa I, Janis JE. Maximizing technological resources in plastic surgery resident education [Review]. J Craniofac Surg 2015;26(8):2264–9.
6. Papas A, Montemurro P, Heden P. Aesthetic training for plastic surgeons: are residents getting enough? [Review]. Aesthet Plast Surg 2018;42(1):327–30.
7. Gardner AK, Grantcharov T, Dunkin BJ. The science of selection: using best practices from industry to improve success in surgery training. J Surg Educ 2018;75(2):278–85.

8. Faucett EA, McCrary HC, Barry JY, et al. High-quality feedback regarding professionalism and communication skills in otolaryngology resident education [Review]. Otolaryngol Head Neck Surg 2018; 158(1):36–42.

9. Musbahi O, Aydin A, Al Omran Y, et al. Current status of simulation in otolaryngology: a systematic review [Review]. J Surg Educ 2017;74(2):203–15.

10. Javia L, Sardesai MG. Physical models and virtual reality simulators in otolaryngology [Review]. Otolaryngol Clin North Am 2017;50(5):875–91.

11. Meara DJ, Coffey ZS. Simulation in craniomaxillofacial training [Review]. Curr Opin Otolaryngol Head Neck Surg 2016;24(4):376–80.

12. Volk MS. Improving team performance through simulation-based learning [Review]. Otolaryngol Clin North Am 2017;50(5):967–87.

13. Wagner N, Fahim C, Dunn K, et al. Otolaryngology residency education: a scoping review on the shift towards competency-based medical education [Review]. Clin Otolaryngol 2017;42(3):564–72.

14. Yeh DH, Fung K, Malekzadeh S, et al. Preparing for residency [Review]. Otolaryngol Clin North Am 2017;50(5):1003–13.

15. Cavel O, Giguere C, Lapointe A, et al. Training: simulating pediatric airway [Review]. Pediatr Clin North Am 2013;60(4):993–1003.

16. Mackay DR. Obtaining accreditation council for graduate medical education approval for international rotations during plastic surgery residency training [Review]. J Craniofac Surg 2015;26(4): 1086–7.

17. Ho T, Bentz M, Brzezienski M, et al. The present status of global mission trips in plastic surgery residency programs [Review]. J Craniofac Surg 2015; 26(4):1088–90.

18. Hau DK, Smart LR, DiPace JI, et al. Global health training among U.S. residency specialties: a systematic literature review [Review]. Med Educ Online 2017;22(1):1270020.

19. Lim R, Thaller S. The role of overseas missions in plastic surgery resident education [Review]. J Craniofac Surg 2015;26(4):1134–5.

20. Tarpada SP, Hsueh WD, Gibber MJ. Resident and student education in otolaryngology: A 10-year update on e-learning [Review]. Laryngoscope 2017; 127(7):E219–24.

21. Jensen RL, Alzhrani G, Kestle JRW, et al. Neurosurgeon as educator: a review of principles of adult education and assessment applied to neurosurgery. J Neurosurg 2017;127:949–57.

22. Kolb D. Experiencial learning: experience as a source of learning and development. New York: Pearson Education, Inc; 1984.

23. Arora A, Lau LY, Awad Z, et al. Virtual reality simulation training in otolaryngology [Review]. Int J Surg 2014;12(2):87–94.

24. Diaz-Siso JR, Plana NM, Stranix JT, et al. Computer simulation and digital resources for plastic surgery psychomotor education [Review]. Plast Reconstr Surg 2016;138(4):730e–8e.

25. Loh CYY, Wang AYL, Tiong VTY, et al. Animal models in plastic and reconstructive surgery simulation-a review [Review]. J Surg Res 2018; 221:232–45.

26. Cingi C, Oghan F. Teaching 3D sculpting to facial plastic surgeons [Review]. Facial Plast Surg Clin North Am 2011;19(4):603–14.

27. VanKoevering KK, Malloy KM. Emerging role of three-dimensional printing in simulation in otolaryngology [Review]. Otolaryngol Clin North Am 2017; 50(5):947–58.

28. Mazza E, Barbarino GG. 3D mechanical modeling of facial soft tissue for surgery simulation [Review]. Facial Plast Surg Clin North Am 2011;19(4):623–37.

29. Piromchai P, Avery A, Laopaiboon M, et al. Virtual reality training for improving the skills needed for performing surgery of the ear, nose or throat [Review]. Cochrane Database Syst Rev 2015;(9): CD010198.

30. Lee AY, Fried MP, Gibber M. Improving rhinology skills with simulation [Review]. Otolaryngol Clin North Am 2017;50(5):893–901.

31. Willaert WI, Aggarwal R, Van Herzeele I, et al. Recent advancements in medical simulation: patient-specific virtual reality simulation [Review]. World J Surg 2012;36(7):1703–12.

32. Bowe SN, Johnson K, Puscas L. Facilitation and debriefing in simulation education [Review]. Otolaryngol Clin North Am 2017;50(5):989–1001.

33. Davis CR, Rosenfield LK. Looking at plastic surgery through Google Glass: part 1. Systematic review of Google Glass evidence and the first plastic surgical procedures [Review]. Plast Reconstr Surg 2015; 135(3):918–28.

34. Sullivan SA, Anderson BM, Pugh CM. Development of technical skills: education, simulation, and maintenance of certification [Review]. J Craniofac Surg 2015;26(8):2270–4.

35. Simmons BJ, Zoghbi Y, Askari M, et al. Significance of objective structured clinical examinations to plastic surgery residency training [Review]. Ann Plast Surg 2017;79(3):312–9.

36. Bhatti NI. Assessment of surgical skills and competency [Review]. Otolaryngol Clin North Am 2017; 50(5):959–65.

37. Gosman A, Mann K, Reid CM, et al. Implementing assessment methods in plastic surgery [Review]. Plast Reconstr Surg 2016;137(3):617e–23e.

38. Labbe M, Young M, Nguyen LHP. Validity evidence as a key marker of quality of technical skill assessment in OTL-HNS [Review]. Laryngoscope 2018; 128(10):2296–300.

Facial Plastic Surgery Journals
Understanding Their Relevance and Getting Published

Ari Hyman, MD[a,*], John Rhee, MD, MPH[b]

KEYWORDS

- Altmetric score • High impact article • H-index • Impact factor • Mendeley readership score

KEY POINTS

- Contemporary scientific journal readership has largely transitioned from primarily print media to an online digital media format, with most articles being read online.
- The movement to distribute pertinent medical knowledge outside the confines of the medical community and capture a wider global readership is now measured by a metric of academic impact and are termed "alternative metrics."
- Common metrics for measuring the digital dissemination that accompanies any given publication are the altmetric score and the Mendeley readership score.
- The impact factor is a metric used for a given scientific journal that is designed to assess a journal's overall scientific quality.
- The number of recent downloads or views is the metric that can be used to assess reader interest.

INTRODUCTION

It can often be confusing to a prospective author as to what makes a manuscript for publication consideration attractive to a particular journal. It is also interesting to consider that much of today's readership has transitioned to digital formats and many articles are increasingly being read online. Furthermore, the Internet and social media's impact on the medical literature has greatly increased exposure of medical knowledge well outside the limits of the scientific community and now impacts the public and the perception of the specialty as a whole. Therefore, understanding a journal's vision and metrics of success and impact can help align the goals of authors and journal editors. The metrics that most substantially impact a journal, and in many ways drive decision-making in terms of what to accept for publication, include citations, number of views or downloads, and social media or public attention that accompanies any given publication (**Fig. 1**). These metrics translate into publications that either in isolation or in combination showcase the best science, serve to educate, and/or frame the most pertinent and contemporary issues relevant to the field of facial plastic surgery. These metrics produce what we call "high-impact" articles, which in turn align with the journal's strategic vision and relevance. This article further defines these guiding metrics with the goal of informing the prospective authors who seek to publish their manuscripts in facial plastic surgery journals.[1]

[a] Facial Plastic and Reconstructive Surgery, 16311 Ventura Boulevard #600, Encino, CA 91436, USA;
[b] Department of Otolaryngology Head and Neck Surgery, Medical College of Wisconsin, 9200 West Wisconsin Avenue, Milwaukee, WI 53226, USA
* Corresponding author.
E-mail address: Arihymanmd@gmail.com

Facial Plast Surg Clin N Am 28 (2020) 477–481
https://doi.org/10.1016/j.fsc.2020.06.006

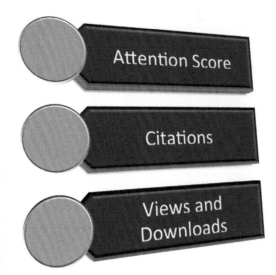

Fig. 1. High-impact article metrics.

ALTMETRIC SCORE AND MENDELEY READER SCORE

An important shift in the paradigm surrounding medical literature is that distribution of medical knowledge is no longer limited to the confines of the academic community. With the use of Internet and social media, discovery and medical information is now reaching a broader audience and the demand from the public for peer-reviewed information has increased. The field of facial plastic surgery, in particular, garners interest from the lay public and there has been a concerted effort by the specialty journals to distribute information by way of social media platforms and other media outlets to increase engagement and to educate the public of scientific trends in the field. For example, *JAMA Facial Plastic Surgery,* which releases weekly "online first" publications, also uses Twitter and Facebook to release evidence-based literature to patients and to the public as a means of increasing engagement and knowledge. This movement to distribute pertinent medical knowledge outside the confines of the medical community, to engage with the public, and to capture a wider global readership is now measured by a metric of academic impact and termed "alternative metrics." Common metrics used include the altmetric score and the Mendeley reader score. The altmetric score of an article is based on mentions from news outlets and multiple social media platforms like Facebook and Twitter, which then generate an "altmetric attention score." The formula for its calculation considers each media channels' impact on potential readers. An article that is mentioned by a news outlet receives a

weight of 8, whereas a mention on Twitter is given a weight of 1.[2] The Altmetric score appears to be the most frequently used metric and is highlighted by most the major journals publishing within our field. An example of a publication that has garnered significant attention and achieved a high altmetric score in the facial plastic literature is an article by Popenko and colleagues[3] from 2017 in *JAMA Facial Plastic Surgery* on the ideal female lip aesthetic and its effect on facial attractiveness. This article was viewed more than 53,000 times, cited 14 times, and has an altmetric score of 497 (**Fig. 2**).[3] Altmetric scores can be quite high, particularly in broader fields such as internal medicine. An article from July 2019 on the ketogenic diet for obesity and diabetes published in *JAMA Internal Medicine* boasts an altmetric score of 1390.[4] To further highlight this point, an article published in *The New England Journal of Medicine* on mortality in Puerto Rico after Hurricane Maria published in 2018 reached an altmetric score of 10,503 (**Fig. 3**).[5]

Another example of a metric that collects and presents digital data is the Mendeley readership score. This particular measure is based on how frequently an article is collected in a user's personal library within the global research community. The geographic locations, specialties of study, and academic ranks of the researchers using these articles are also considered in its calculation. Journals are exceedingly aware of the shifting paradigm from engagement limited to a select few within a small scientific field to a global readership with potentially limitless engagement. To highlight this point, many journals now display on their Web site how an article is performing in terms of these metrics. For example, the *Plastic and Reconstructive Surgery Journal* Web site has a built in "Article Metrics" tool that allows the user to browse the number of views, citations, and downloads, as well as the altmetric score and Mendeley readership score for each featured journal article. The *Aesthetic Surgery Journal* readily offers readers the number of views, citations and the altmetric score of all of its articles through its "view metrics" tab on the journal's Web site. *Otolaryngology–Head and Neck Surgery* journal, too, offers these same metrics.

CITATION AND IMPACT FACTOR

Increasing emphasis on the importance of evidence-based medicine has brought about increased pressures on the academic community to produce peer-reviewed manuscripts. Citation metrics are likely familiar to many within the scientific community. A common metric that has been

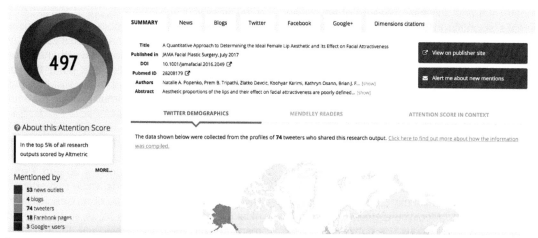

Fig. 2. A quantitative approach to determining the ideal female lip aesthetic and its affect on facial attractiveness: an example of a high altmetric score from the facial plastic literature. (*From* Popenko NA, Tripathi PB, et al. A Quantitative Approach to Determining the Ideal Female Lip Aesthetic and Its Effect on Facial Attractiveness. JAMA Facial Plast Surg. 2017;19(4):261–267. https://doi.org/10.1001/jamafacial.2016.2049.)

shown to impact promotion or grant funding for the individual author is the Hirsch-index or "H-Index." The H-index takes into account the number of articles published by an author and the citations to those papers as a means of evaluating a given author's impact. The citation benchmark percentile and field-weighted citation impact are other metrics that consider the impact of a given publication in terms of its citations. The citation benchmark compares the number of citations per article with other articles published over the past 18 months within the same discipline. The field-weighted citation impact reflects how well an article has been cited over a 3-year window in comparison with articles within the same field published within a similar timeframe. A field-weighted citation impact greater than 1.0 describes an article that is cited more than what is expected of the mean.[6]

The Impact Factor (IF) is an annual metric, calculated by Thomson Reuters, given to a scientific journal that is in part to assess a journal's relative scientific quality and influence. The IF of a journal is calculated by counting all of the citations to every article published in a journal divided by the number of "substantial" articles (original research, long reviews, special communications) published in that specific journal during the 2 preceding years. In many ways, IF has become a

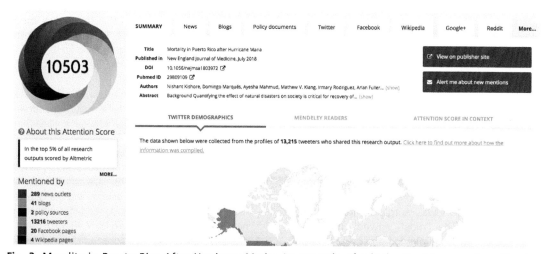

Fig. 3. Morality in Puerto Rico After Hurricane Maria: An example of a high altmetric score from literature outside of facial plastic surgery. (*From* Kishore N, Marqués D, Mahmud A, et al. Mortality in Puerto Rico after hurricane Maria. N Engl J Med. 2018;379(2):162–70. https://doi.org/10.1056/NEJMsa1803972 Epub 2018 May 29.)

fundamental and universal measure of any given journal's scientific influence.[7] Impact factors for specialized disciplines like facial plastic surgery typically have a lower score than less specialized fields and general medical journals. This is in part because clinically based fields like facial plastic surgery often experience a lag in terms of its citation frequency as opposed to the basic sciences that tend to be cited more frequently since the knowledge and reporting cycle runs on a faster pace in the basic science literature.[1] The most prominent plastic surgery and facial plastic surgery journals range in IF from 2.0 to 4.0. By comparison, the IF of a journal such as *The New England Journal of Medicine* is greater than 70.0. Highly citable publications, or publications that factor into the calculation of a journal's IF are therefore an important consideration for medical journals reviewing any manuscript for submission as these in turn contribute to a journal's overall IF standing. Journals take note of what are the most cited recent publications, and in this era of digitalization, often highlight those publications on a journal's Web site or online portal. For example, on *JAMA Facial Plastic Surgery's* homepage, the "most cited" article of the past 3 years is about standardized cosmesis and health nasal outcomes surveys, being viewed 2649 times, along with its 18 citations.[8] The journal's IF too is commonly highlighted on a journals homepage. The importance of citation metrics will likely persist into the future and potential citability is a strong consideration when scientific manuscripts are reviewed.

DOWNLOADS AND VIEWERSHIP

Apart from a manuscript's potential citability, another area of interest for journals are articles or publications that are likely to draw interest from its readership for reasons such as clinical applicability. With articles being increasingly read online, Web sites now often list the number of recent downloads or views as a reflection of a particular publication's popularity. The number of recent downloads is the metric that can be used to assess overall reader interest. Articles that increase readership or draw interest from current readership come in any form but are often clinically significant or are educationally focused. Examples of this in the facial plastic surgery literature include in-depth topic reviews, surgical vignettes, or opinion pieces. The "most viewed" article on *JAMA Facial Plastic Surgery's* homepage is about the association between social media and photograph editing use, self-esteem, and cosmetic surgery acceptance, having been viewed more than

4500 times with an altmetric score of 160 and 0 citations.[9] This metric, the number of views or downloads, is another measure of a journal's value to its readership. The metrics associated with the aforementioned article exemplifies the point that an article that may be important to the viewership of a subspecialty medical journal may or may not correlate with citations. *JAMA Facial Plastic Surgery* "Surgical Pearls," are a great example of a highly viewed publication format. The surgical pearl on nonsurgical rhinoplasty had more than 3000 views, an altmetric score of 20 and 2 citations, reflecting its educational value to readers.[10] Recognizing the unique nature of subspecialty surgical journals and its desire to be an educational resource for their readership is an important concept for prospective authors to understand.

SUMMARY

It can often be confusing to the author as to what makes a submission for publication "publishable" or attractive to a journal. Much of today's readership has transitioned to digital formats with many articles now read online. The Internet and social media's impact on the medical literature has greatly increased exposure of medical knowledge well outside the limits of the scientific community and now impacts the public and the perception of the specialty. Therefore, it is useful to understand a journal's needs and vision in order to successfully contribute one's work by making efforts to connect with the important metrics of impact or success. These metrics (citations, view popularity, and public attention) often influence the editor's selection of articles for publication. These metrics translate into publications that either in isolation or in combination showcase the best science, serve to educate, and/or frame the most pertinent and contemporary issues relevant to the field of facial plastic surgery.

REFERENCES

1. Rhee JS. High-impact articles—citations, downloads, and altmetric score. JAMA Facial Plast Surg 2015;17(5):323–4.
2. Ruan, Qing, Zhao, et al. Alternative metrics of scholarly output. Plast Reconstr Surg 2018;141(3):801–9.
3. Popenko NA, Tripathi PB, Devcic Z, et al. A quantitative approach to determining the ideal female lip aesthetic and its effect on facial attractiveness. JAMA Facial Plast Surg 2017;19(4):261–7.
4. Joshi S, Ostfeld RJ, McMacken M. The ketogenic diet for obesity and diabetes—enthusiasm outpaces evidence. JAMA Intern Med 2019. https://doi.org/10.1001/jamainternmed.2019.2633.

5. Kishore N, Marqués D, Mahmud A, et al. Mortality in Puerto Rico after hurricane Maria. N Engl J Med 2018;379(2):162–70.

6. García-Pérez, Miguel A. The hirsch h index in a non-mainstream area: methodology of the behavioral sciences in Spain. Span J Psychol 2009;12(2):833–49.

7. Grzybowski A, Patryn R. Impact factor: universalism and reliability of assessment. Clin Dermatol 2017; 35(3):331–4.

8. Saltychev M, Kandathil CK, Abdelwahab M, et al. Psychometric properties of the standardized cosmesis and health nasal outcomes survey: item response theory analysis. JAMA Facial Plast Surg 2018;20(6):519–21.

9. Chen J, Ishii M, Bater KL, et al. Association between the use of social media and photograph editing applications, self-esteem, and cosmetic surgery acceptance. JAMA Facial Plast Surg 2019. https://doi.org/10.1001/jamafacial.2019. 0328.

10. Kontis TC. Nonsurgical rhinoplasty. JAMA Facial Plast Surg 2017;19(5):430–1.

Recognizing, Managing, and Guiding the Patient Through Complications in Facial Plastic Surgery

Phillip R. Langsdon, MD[a,b,*], Ronald J. Schroeder II, MD[c,1]

KEYWORDS

- Complications • Neuromodulators • Dermal fillers • Laser resurfacing • Infection • Hematoma
- Nerve injury

KEY POINTS

- Understanding of facial muscle anatomy and proper patient education to aid in handling inadvertent ptosis with neuromodulators.
- Understanding dermal filler emergency, treatment protocol, and staff training is essential to respond to vascular occlusion with dermal fillers.
- Proper patient selection and laser settings can minimize risk with pigment changes and scarring from laser resurfacing procedures.
- Early identification of postsurgical complications may minimize long-term sequelae.
- Frequent communication between patient and surgeon/staff helps recognize early complications and aids in patient satisfaction.

INTRODUCTION

Throughout our training and careers as facial plastic surgeons we master relevant anatomy, facial analysis, patient evaluation, and multiple procedure techniques in order to maximize our outcomes and reduce our complication rates. But no matter how proficient we may be, complications are periodically unavoidable. They may occur from multifactorial reasons (surgical technique, medical comorbidities, medications, poor compliance, etc.). In this article, we will discuss how to reduce, recognize, and manage these complications.

CONTENT

Patient Evaluation

Complication prevention starts during the initial consultation. The patient is analyzed to determine what procedures can be offered to address the patient's concerns. This is followed by a discussion of the procedure, postoperative care, alternatives, risks, complications, limitations, and potential need for additional treatment. It is stressed that perfection is not promised and asymmetries are pointed out. The patient is photographed in 3-dimensional (to point out asymmetries), point flash (to provide crisp outlines), and bounce flash photography (to demonstrate surface irregularities

[a] The Langsdon Clinic, 7499 Poplar Pike, Germantown, TN, USA; [b] Department of Otolaryngology–Head and Neck Surgery, University of Tennessee Health Science Center, Memphis, TN, USA; [c] Midwest Facial Plastic Surgery, Woodbury, MN, USA
[1] Present address: 2080 Woodwinds Drive, Suite 220, Woodbury, MN 55125.
* Corresponding author.
E-mail address: langsdon@bellsouth.net

Facial Plast Surg Clin N Am 28 (2020) 483–491
https://doi.org/10.1016/j.fsc.2020.06.007
1064-7406/20/© 2020 Elsevier Inc. All rights reserved.

and volume issues). Photography is vitally important so that we can verify changes and prove pre-existing conditions.

Often times a patient may not understand what a particular procedure is designed to enhance and what cannot be accomplished with that procedure. For instance, a procedure that is designed to treat sagging facial skin and muscle will not make the skin surface smoother or restore volume loss. Perhaps a patient may need facial resurfacing for surface irregularities and/or injectable fillers for volume loss. Patients must understand these issues and willingly accept the reality of their condition and the limitations of the treatment selected.

Patients often expect that a single procedure is going to give them the perfect result they are imagining. But in reality, we understand that there are many factors that may not make this possible. Improvement, rather than perfection, is a realistic expectation. If a potential patient does not accept this distinction, as well as the reality of what a procedure will and will not accomplish, and what adjunctive procedures may be necessary, we will not treat the patient. Patient satisfaction is often the difference between the expectations you establish as the surgeon and what the patient perceives. Therefore, it is of paramount importance to emphasize a set of realistic expectations and determine if the patient will accept these realities.

Identifying patients with unrealistic expectations who may become problem patients postoperatively is one of the most challenging aspects of our field. One of the simplest ways of determining this is to ask why a patient desires to have a procedure done. Many patients can easily verbalize their motives and goals, but those who struggle to clarify their goals should cause some provider concern. In addition, patients who are overanalytical may hyperfocus on subtle irregularities that are virtually imperceptible to anyone else. No matter how much you discuss the realistic objectives with these types of patients, they have a high likelihood of being dissatisfied with their result. This then leads into the question of whether or not the patient falls into the category of body dysmorphic disorder (BDD). BDD is a mental disorder in the obsessive-compulsive spectrum where patients display excessive concern with minor or wholly nonexistent defects in physical appearance.[1] This disorder can be easily screened for by having a patient fill out a BDD questionnaire (**Fig. 1**). Patients with BDD will often answer most, if not all, questions in the affirmative, which should prompt the surgeon to have a discussion with the patient about working with a psychiatrist. This is a delicate topic as many patients do not realize they have a problem and may be offended or upset at the suggestion. Our approach is to diplomatically state that we feel that we need the evaluation and assistance of a psychological professional before we can consider agreeing to treat the patient. This is not a promise to treat but only for further consideration.

It is also important at this stage to distinguish between what is a normal side effect of the procedure (ie, bruising, swelling, etc.) and what is considered a complication (ie, hematoma, infection, etc.). A patient who may have normal post-procedure bruising and swelling may be perceive that as a "complication" if they were not adequately educated on what to expect. Even when properly educated, many patients need professional reassurance and follow-up to help them know what is normal. Otherwise a patient may be very dissatisfied with their care even in the setting of an excellent result. On the other hand, a patient who was properly informed but develops a real complication that is recognized and managed in a timely manner may have a much higher level of satisfaction. Informing the patient of the relative risk of a complication and how it is recognized and managed establishes a sense of trust during the consultation process. Some surgeons may be hesitant to go in much detail about surgical risks, as this may deter a patient from proceeding with surgery, but most of the patients recognize and accept the risk of complication if they trust their surgeon will take care of them.

Lastly, as with any consult it is imperative to obtain a complete medical, surgical, and medication history. Multiple risk factors may be identified that can affect bleeding, wound healing, and infection. If these factors are identified it is important to share this information with the patient and what can be done to mitigate the associated risk (modify procedural technique, hold medication, etc.). For surgical procedures, preoperative medical evaluation, blood work, and electrocardiogram may be recommended for select patients. Taking the time to adequately prepare a patient for a procedure can sometimes prevent complications. It has been my practice for invasive surgical procedures to obtain a broad battery of laboratory work in order to determine adequate blood counts, blood clotting ability, general health, as well as the presence of communicable diseases that can either infect staff or interfere with the patients healing capacity.

Injectables

Neuromodulators and dermal fillers have quickly become common aesthetic procedures. This is due in large part to their effectiveness and low

Are you worried about how you look? Examples of areas of concern include: skin (for example; scars, wrinkles, redness), the shape of your nose, mouth jaw or lips: Please list specific areas_____
_____.

Do you deliberately check your features in the mirror multiple times each day?	Yes / No
Do you avoid mirrors, photos, or videos of yourself?	Yes / No
Do you feel like your features are unattractive?	Yes / No
Do your features cause you a lot of distress?	Yes / No
Do your features cause you to avoid situations or activities?	Yes / No
Do your features preoccupy your thoughts?	Yes / No
Do your features have an effect on your relationships?	Yes / No
Do your features interfere with your social life?	Yes / No
Do you feel your appearance is the most important aspect of who you are?	Yes / No

Fig. 1. Body dysmorphic disorder questionnaire.

complication profile. As a result, there are many injectors serving as providers with a variety of background and training. Those with less experience or poor training with facial anatomy may place their patients at increased risk of complications.

Bruising and swelling

When counseling patients who are interested in a neuromodulator or dermal filler, we mention that a common risk is bruising and swelling. As previously mentioned, these are potential side effects and not complications; however, patients often have an expectation of no visible side effects because injections are "minimally invasive." Patients should be counseled that certain areas are more prone to edema and ecchymosis, particularly the lips and tear troughs, but that this can occur at any injection site. Hematoma is exceedingly rare but certainly possible, especially in patients on anticoagulants. Sometimes prominent vessels can be identified and avoided during injection. There have been reports that 25-gauge or larger cannulas may reduce the risk of vessel injury.[2] However, there are concerns with accuracy of filler placement with some cannulas. Ecchymosis can often be identified immediately after removal of the needle or cannula, in which case holding pressure for 1 to 2 minutes may prevent it from enlarging. However, we have seen bruising occur days after injections. It is also important to educate patients that applying ice, avoiding strenuous activity, and keeping their head elevated for about 24 hours may reduce the risk of ecchymosis and edema after the procedure.

If a patient develops significant edema or ecchymosis, reassurance that it will resolve is important. Short-term edema can be managed conservatively with cold compresses, but if it persists a short course of an oral steroid may help. Long-term edema is rare but has been reported in patients who had tear trough filler years prior. Fortunately, this has been shown to be effectively treated with hyaluronidase.[3] It is uncommon for a patient to have a significant amount of ecchymosis after an injection, but intense pulsed light (IPL) and broadband light (BBL) may reduce ecchymosis within hours after treatment.[4] Arnica and bromelain have been used both orally and topically for reduction of postprocedure ecchymosis; however, there is currently insufficient evidence to support these claims.[5]

Infection

Any procedure that breaks the skin has a risk of infection. Fortunately, this is very rare with neuromodulators and dermal fillers, as long aseptic technique is used. Any patient with an active skin infection (viral, bacterial, fungal) should not be injected until the infection resolves. Patients with a history of herpes simplex virus may be pretreated with an antiviral medication (acyclovir, valacyclovir, or famciclovir) or treated when symptomatic after injection.[6] Bacterial infections typically present as worsening erythema and pain, and they should be treated with oral antibiotics appropriate for skin flora (cephalexin or amoxicillin). If the patient has a history of methicillin-resistant *Staphylococcus aureus*, then consider starting clindamycin or a tetracycline antibiotic.[7] If a bacterial infection is not treated early, then it may progress to an abscess necessitating surgical drainage.

Neuromodulators

Neuromodulators are all derivatives of botulinum toxin, which prevents acetylcholine release at the neuromuscular junction leading to muscle weakness. As a result, complications related to botulinum toxin therapy are related to unintended paralysis of nearby muscles. The most troublesome is the levator palpebrae muscle that may run deep to the lateral corrugator muscle. Levator paralysis leads to upper eyelid ptosis that is not only cosmetically undesirable but can also lead to vision difficulties.[8] In addition, inadvertent paralysis of the extraocular muscles or lacrimal gland may result in strabismus, diplopia, or dry eye syndrome.[9] These complications can result from injection technique, atypical anatomy, or inadvertent pressure on the face causing the toxin to spread. However, eyelid ptosis can occur even in ideal situations with a perfect injection process. Therefore, the development of an eyelid ptosis should be discussed with the patient and he/she should understand that it can and does occur even in the best of situations and even when it did not occur with prior treatments. A safe injection technique is to avoid injecting beyond the medial one-third of the eyebrow and inject superficially and slowly immediately under the dermis. It is important to educate the patient to avoid any pressure on their face for 48 hours, including sleeping on their face, lying prone on a massage table, scuba diving, or even getting on an airplane. If a patient develops upper eyelid ptosis, apraclonidine drops may be used to activate Mueller muscle until the toxin wears off in 3 to 4 months.[10]

Neuromodulation is otherwise very safe, and expert injectors understand the balance between the action and counteraction of various muscle groups. Injection of the glabella and crow's feet areas can be used as a "chemical brow lift" by creating unopposed action of the frontalis. However, some patients wish to have their forehead rhytids improved, and brow ptosis and/or a shiny "frozen" forehead may occur when treating the forehead in some patients. It is important to discuss the limits of forehead injection with the patient before injecting the frontalis so that they will understand the potential downside to obtaining a total resolution of forehead lines. Often times a cosmetically pleasing result can be produced by injecting a small dosage (4–6 units) across the frontalis that results in weakness instead of paralysis of the frontalis that improves the forehead rhytids without producing an unnatural appearance.

Injection limited to the medial frontalis can result in a peaked lateral or "spock" eyebrows.[11] Fortunately, injecting 1 to 2 units a few centimeters above the peaked eyebrow can improve this condition.

Dermal fillers

There are a several dermal filler products available including hyaluronic acid (HA), calcium hydroxylapatite, polymethyl methacrylate, poly-L-lactic acid, collagen, and silicon. Each of these products has their own risk and benefit profile, but HA fillers are by far the most common because of their versatility and their reversibility with hyaluronidase. Regardless of the product used, irregularities, asymmetry, and lumps can occur. These lumps may appear in areas of thin soft-tissue coverage such as the lips and tear troughs. Firm massage may help disperse the product, otherwise consider reversing with hyaluronidase when the acute edema has resolved.[12]

The most severe acute complication is vascular compromise from either intraarterial injection or vessel compression. Aspirating before each injection, injecting small aliquots filler, or use of blunt cannulas may reduce the risk of vascular compromise. Presentation can vary from immediate blanching of skin to delayed skin changes eventually leading to necrosis or loss of vision.[13] Early identification and treatment may help prevent permanent sequelae. Large amounts of hyaluronidase should be immediately injected regardless of the type of filler used because of its edema-reducing benefits and theoretic advantage in reducing the occluding vessel pressure.[14] In addition, warm compresses, massaging the area, and the application of topical nitroglycerin paste may help.[15] Aspirin and intravenous prostaglandins have been suggested, but their efficacy has not yet been proved.[16] If skin necrosis is evident, the patient should be started on an antibiotic and local debridement and wound care performed as needed.[12] A change in vision warrants the immediate consultation with an ophthalmologist. Some have suggested the intraorbital injection of hyaluronidase.

Nodules and granulomas are long-term complications that can occur with any dermal filler. There is some debate regarding HA fillers whether nodules are more commonly seen with certain products or if it is related to injection technique. Regardless of the cause, first-line treatment is intralesional injection with hyaluronidase. If the nodule persists, then intralesional steroid injection may help.[17] If intralesional injections fail, then direct excision may be performed.

Resurfacing Procedures

Skin resurfacing techniques traditionally involve the use of a controlled depth of injury with mechanical, chemical, or light-based tools to remove the surface of the skin in varying depths, thus stimulating the reepithelialization process and possibly generating new dermal collagen and elastin. Chemical peels initiate resurfacing by chemically injuring the skin surface. Dermabrasion stimulates resurfacing by mechanically removing the skin surface. Laser technology removes the skin surface by thermal injury. Greater results are typically seen with greater depth of skin insult and removal. However, the greater the depth of insult, the longer the recovery period, and the increased risk of healing side effects and complications.

The CO_2 laser continues to be an excellent tool for aggressive skin resurfacing. This laser can be used in either a fractionated or nonfractionated manner. Fractional lasers have been shown to have a lower rate of complications but may require multiple treatments to achieve the same results of a nonfractionated ablative laser.[18] Although ablative nonfractionated lasers are potentially more effective in reducing wrinkles, there is more long-term redness, healing, posttreatment pigment changes, and a higher risk of scarring when used in high settings, depending on skin type and sensitivity, facial location, and thickness. As a result, fractional CO_2 laser is currently a commonly used tool in order to reduce risk and recovery time. There are other skin resurfacing technologies, including plasma, radiofrequency, and microultrasound, but there remains a lack of evidence of the efficacy of these modalities. Regardless of the technology used, any time the skin is insulted, the skin is at risk for pigment changes, scarring, infection, and contact dermatitis.

Infection

Skin is our first line of defense against infection, so naturally damaging the skin with resurfacing techniques increases the risk of infection. The presence of an active infection site may increase the risk of an infection spreading over the treated field. Reactivation of herpes simplex virus and herpes zoster virus can occur after skin resurfacing. If a patient has a history of these infections, then it may be helpful to institute prophylactic treatment with antivirals. Some practitioners suggest placing all skin resurfacing patients on antivirals.

Bacterial infections are rare, but usually caused by poor hygiene. It is important to counsel patients on how to care for their skin after the procedure including frequent gentle cleaning and debridement with pressurized water (shower or

sink nozzle) and liberal use of petroleum-based ointment. Patients should avoid picking at any crusting or flaking, as fingers are common sources of unwanted bacteria. Infection should be suspected in patients with worsening edema, erythema, pain, and possibly fever. Sometimes this can be difficult to identify after skin resurfacing, but we have a low threshold for initiating empirical antibiotic therapy.

Pigment changes

When resurfaced skin heals, the inflammation from the healing leaves the skin erythematous for a period of time. This is a normal part of the recovery, but it may be prolonged in some patients. Reassurance will help in many situations, but if prolonged beyond a few weeks we may start our patients on a daily application of hydrocortisone cream. We use 1% for mild cases and 2.5% for more intense erythema.

Patients with Fitzpatrick skin type III or higher are at increased risk of both postprocedure hyperpigmentation and hypopigmentation. With the use of fractional lasers, this is less common.[19] Although seen more frequently with an ablative CO_2 laser treatment, aggressive laser settings and multiple passes in patients with fractional lasers or in some patients with very sensitive skin may also disrupt melanogenesis leading to hypopigmentation. Patients with darker skin types can be pretreated with hydroquinone to inactivate tyrosine kinase, thereby hopefully decreasing risk of hyperpigmentation.[20] If hyperpigmentation occurs, treatment with PDL, IPL, BBL, or retreatment at different settings than the initial resurfacing technique may help.[21]

It should also be mentioned that other skin treatments such as with an IPL machine used for something as simple as hair removal may incite hyperpigmentation changes in certain genetic skin types.[22]

Contact dermatitis may be due to an irritant or an allergy and can occur at any time during the postprocedure course of any type of resurfacing. Early on, this may be difficult to distinguish from an infection, but contact dermatitis may often present as symmetric erythema and edema (**Fig. 2**). It is important to educate patients that resurfaced skin is very sensitive and may react to various topical creams, lotions, and cleansers even if it is a product they have used for several years.[23] The offending agent should be discontinued immediately and the contact dermatitis treated with topical $1/4$% acetic acid soaks applied twice a day, an oral antihistamine, and 1% topical hydrocortisone cream applied twice a day.

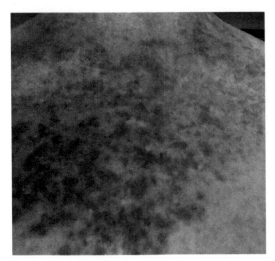

Fig. 2. Contact dermatitis after fractional CO2 laser of the neck and chest.

Scarring

Scarring that occurs from skin resurfacing can result from overly sensitive skin type, aggressive resurfacing, or from infection. Areas of thin skin (ie, neck and eyelids) are more susceptible to scarring.[24] However, scarring may occur in areas that are aggressively treated for deep rhytids, such as in the perioral area of patients with deep regional wrinkles who insist on aggressive treatment. In most instances scarring is cosmetic; however, significant scar contraction of the thin eyelid skin can lead to functional issues such as ectropion or lagophthalmos. We are cautious in patients with history of a subciliary blepharoplasty incision, scleral show, large globes, and lower eyelid laxity.[25] The presence of these conditions does not mean these patients cannot be treated. However, we proceed with caution, good patient education, lowered expectations, and a less aggressive treatment. In spite of all the preparation and precautions, sometimes complications such as ectropion occur. Most situations within our patient population and under our treatment protocols are usually self-limiting. We institute globe protection protocols with early taping and lubrication. If necessary, a lid suspension and tightening procedure will be used.

In areas where deeper treatment is indicated such as in deep perioral rhytids, we carefully monitor the patient's postoperative healing course. If there is any delay in healing, we may begin topical steroids and increase the frequency of clinical evaluations.

Treatment options for scarring from resurfacing are essentially the same as those for surgical scarring. Early treatment of hypertrophic scars typically consists of topical 2.5% hydrocortisone cream.[26] We progress to intralesional steroid injections as necessary. In addition, intralesional injections of chemotherapeutic medications (5-fluorouracil, interferon, bleomycin, etc.) have also been shown to be effective.[27] Lasers (CO2, Er:YAG, Argon) may reduce hypertrophic scars in some situations. If conservative treatment fails, then direct excision may be considered.

Surgical Complications

Thorough understanding of surgical anatomy and good technique is obviously necessary in reducing risk of complications. However, no matter how meticulous we are in our technique, surgical complications will occur. Early identification is critical, so evaluating the patient before discharge and maintaining frequent communication after discharge by surgeon or staff can aid in recognizing complications in a timely manner.

Hematoma

Intraoperative and postoperative bleeding is a risk in every surgery. Hematoma formation is one of the most common postsurgical complications but can be minimized with meticulous surgical hemostasis; proper patient selection; and the cessation of all medications, herbs, and vitamins that may cause bleeding 2 weeks before surgery. We review the patient's medications and provide them with a "do not take" list (medications, herbs, vitamins, and red wine) well before surgery in order to ensure they are not unwittingly taking anything that may interfere with clotting.

We live in an era when the use of mood-altering medications is commonplace. Many of these medications increase bleeding, and some patients are depend on these medications and are unable to stop them before surgery.[28] The use of tranexamic acid in our local injection has proved helpful in cutting down bleeding in these and all patients.[29] Depending on the procedure, drains and pressure dressings may help to reduce the risk of early postoperative hematoma formation. Postoperatively, it is important to counsel patients again on the importance of avoiding head movement, bending over, or any strenuous activity that could stimulate late onset bleeding.

In the early postoperative period, small hematomas can often be expressed through incision lines. Large hematomas, although rare in our practice, may need evacuation and intraoperative hemostasis. Delayed hematomas can occur up to 2 weeks postoperatively and can often be managed with needle aspiration.

Skin necrosis

Skin necrosis can occur in any surgery where a skin flap is elevated or arterial supply is disrupted.

Flap necrosis might occur at the distal ends of flaps where blood supply is most tenuous,[30] this would most commonly be an issue in tobacco users. Caution should be exercised in patients with tobacco use, diabetes, collagen vascular disease, or Raynaud disease. Patients with generalized atherosclerotic vascular disease are also at increased risk. Although all the abovementioned conditions, if not severe, are not necessarily absolute contraindications to surgery, we exercise caution. Our facelift flaps may be shorter than might be used in a healthy patient, and we might decline to place an external incision in a rhinoplasty case in a known patient with Raynaud or lupus if, in the case of a patient with lupus, an antinuclear antibody (ANA) level obtained in their preop examination is high or if the patient with Raynaud disease is a smoker. In patients with elevated antinuclear antibodies, we may delay surgery until levels decline to 1:80.

Tobacco users might be counseled to reduce or discontinue use but this is rarely effective. We may often limit our skin undermining in light smokers, controlled diabetics, or those with inactive collagen vascular disease.

Skin necrosis is often suspected early by duskiness or ecchymosis of the distal flap (**Fig. 3**). If this is detected, then topical nitroglycerin ointment 4 to 6 applications daily may help.[31] Patients should be instructed to make sure the skin is clean before each application. It is important to educate the patient that these areas will have delayed wound healing compared with the rest of the flap. Any eschar formation can be managed with application of hydrogen peroxide at home and in-office debridement as indicated.

Infection

Postsurgical infections are very rare. Antibiotic prophylaxis can be used routinely and should cover *Staphylococcus* and *Streptococcus*. If an early cellulitis develops, we have a high index of suspicion for methicillin-resistant *S aureus*, and we place the patient on a broader spectrum antibiotic with appropriate coverage. Abscess formation is treated as soon as possible with a small incision and drainage in order to prevent spread of the infection along dissection planes (**Fig. 4**). These infections can usually be treated without permanent sequela.

Nerve injury

Nerve injury may be sensory or motor. Sensory reduction is common in most surgeries and not

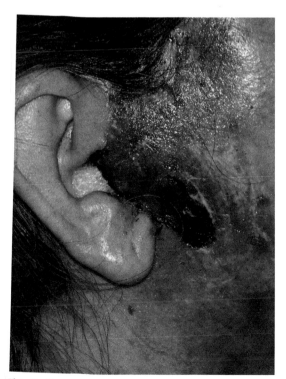

Fig. 3. Flap necrosis 16 days after facelift. Patient was later discovered to have a hypercoagulation condition.

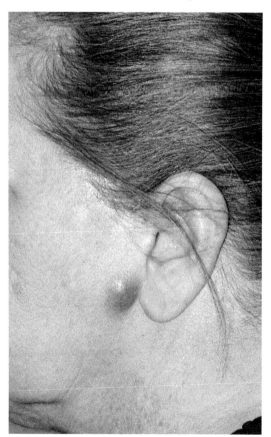

Fig. 4. Suture abscess 12 years after facelift. Suture was removed and patient placed on an antibiotic.

considered a complication, rather a normal consequence of surgery that requires only patient reassurance. Facial motor nerve injury is extremely uncommon but will be evident in the immediate postop period. It is important to reassure the patient at this time that this is likely due to local anesthetic or stretch injury and should resolve. This may resolve in a matter of hours to days or sometimes months.

Injury to the frontal branch of the facial nerve is the most troublesome in facial plastic surgery. If there is significant frontal branch weakness limiting eye closure, it is important to protect the cornea by maintaining hydration with eye drops and/or lubricant, as well as taping the eye shut during sleep. Frontal nerve injury from cautery or stretching can take months to a full year for recovery. Postoperative brow balance can be improved with botulinum toxin neuromodulation of the opposing frontal muscle. Buccal branch weakness can be seen with SMAS deep undermining, but this is not necessarily related to the extent of undermining. Weakness usually resolves over time but can take several months.

SUMMARY

Complications are possible and will occur with every procedure we perform. It is best to try to reduce the risk of complications through proper evaluation, appropriate procedural technique, patient education, and close postoperative monitoring. However, even in the best of circumstances complications will occur. Recognizing and treating complications as early as possible can often reduce long-term consequences. A close patient-physician relationship with ongoing support is important in order to obtain the optimal outcome.

DISCLOSURE

The authors have nothing to disclose.

REFERENCES

1. Hong K, Nezgovorova V, Hollander E. New perspectives in the treatment of body dysmorphic disorder. F1000Res 2018;7:361.
2. Pavicic T, Webb KL, Frnak K, et al. Arterial wall penetration forces in needle versus Cannulas. Plast Reconstr Surg 2019;143(3):504e–12e.
3. Iverson SM, Patel RM. Dermal filler-associated malar edema: Treatment of a persistent adverse effect. Orbit 2017;36(6):473–5.
4. Narurkar V. Post filler ecchymosis resolution with intense pulsed light. J Drugs Dermatol 2018; 17(11):1184–5.
5. Ho D, Jagdeo J, Waldorf HA. Is there a role for arnica and bromelain in prevention of post-procedure ecchymosis or edema? A systematic review of the literature. Dermatol Surg 2016;42(4): 445–63.
6. De Boulle K. Management of complications after implantation of fillers. J Cosmet Dermatol 2004;3:2–15.
7. De Boulle K, Heydenrych I. Patient factors influencing dermal filler complications: prevention, assessment, and treatment. Clin Cosmet Investig Dermatol 2015;8:205–14.
8. Sorensen EP, Urman C. Cosmetic complications: rare and serious events following botulinum toxin and soft tissue filler administration. J Drugs Dermatol 2015;14(5):486–91.
9. Carruthers J, Fournier N, Kerscher M, et al. The convergence of medicine and neurotoxins: A focus on botulinum toxin type A and its application in aesthetic medicine–a global, evidence-based botulinum toxin consensus education initiative: part II: Incorporating botulinum toxin into aesthetic clinical practice. Dermatol Surg 2013;39:510–25.
10. Scheinfeld N. The use of apraclonidine eyedrops to treat ptosis after the administration of botulinum toxin to the upper face. Dermatol Online J 2005; 11(1):9.
11. Carruthers J, Carruthers A. Complications of botulinum toxin type A. Facial Plast Surg Clin North Am 2007;15(1):51–4.
12. Kim JH, Ahn DK, Jeong HS, et al. Treatment algorithm of complications after filler injection: based on wound healing process. J Korean Med Sci 2014;29(Suppl 3):S176–82.
13. Sclafani AP, Fagien S. Treatment of injectable soft tissue filler complications. Dermatol Surg 2009;35: 1672–80.
14. Dayan SH, Arkins JP, Mathison CC. Management of impending necrosis associated with soft tissue filler injections. J Drugs Dermatol 2011;10:1007–12.
15. Urdiales-Gálvez F, Delgado NE, Figueiredo V, et al. Treatment of soft tissue filler complications: expert consensus recommendations. Aesthet Plast Surg 2018;42(2):498–510.
16. Kim SG, Kim YJ, Lee SI, et al. Salvage of nasal skin in a case of venous compromise after hyaluronic acid filler injection using prostaglandin E. Dermatol Surg 2011;37:1817–9.
17. Sperling B, Bachmann F, Hartmann V, et al. The current state of treatment of adverse reactions to injectable fillers. Dermatol Surg 2010;36:1895–904.
18. Chwalek J, Goldberg DJ. Ablative skin resurfacing. Curr Probl Dermatol 2011;42:40–7.
19. Tan KL, Kurniawati C, Gold MH. Low risk of postinflammatory hyperpigmentation in skin types 4 and 5 after treatment with fractional CO2 laser device. J Drugs Dermatol 2008;7(8):774–7.

20. Goldman MP. The use of hydroquinone with facial laser resurfacing. J Cutan Laser Ther 2000;2(2):73–7.
21. Park JH, Kim JI, Kim WS. Treatment of persistent facial postinflammatory hyperpigmentation with novel pulse-in-pulse mode intense pulsed light. Dermatol Surg 2016;42(2):218–24.
22. Fang L, Gold MH, Huang L. Melasma-like hyperpigmentation induced by intense pulsed light in Chinese individuals. J Cosmet Laser Ther 2014;16(6):296–302.
23. Lowe NJ, Lask G, Griffin ME. Laser skin resurfacing. Pre- and posttreatment guidelines. Dermatol Surg 1995;21(12):1017–9.
24. Avram MM, Tope WD, Yu T, et al. Hypertrophic scarring of the neck following ablative fractional carbon dioxide laser resurfacing. Lasers Surg Med 2009; 41(3):185–8.
25. Ramsdell WM. Fractional CO_2 laser resurfacing complications. Semin Plast Surg 2012;26(3):137 40.
26. Issa MC, Kassuga LE, Chevrand NS, et al. Topical delivery of triamcinolone via skin pretreated with ablative radiofrequency: a new method of hypertrophic scar treatment. Int J Dermatol 2013; 52(3):367–70.
27. Darougheh A, Asilian A, Shariati F. Intralesional triamcinolone alone or in combination with 5-fluorouracil for the treatment of keloid and hypertrophic scars. Clin Exp Dermatol 2009;34(2):219–23.
28. Barbui C, Andretta M, De Vitis G, et al. Antidepressant drug prescription and risk of abnormal bleeding: a case-control study. J Clin Psychopharmacol 2009;29(1):33–8.
29. Couto RA, Charafeddine A, Sinclair NR. Local Infiltration of tranexamic acid with local anesthetic reduces intraoperative facelift bleeding: a preliminary report. Aesthet Surg J 2019;40(6):587–93.
30. Gillman GS. Face lift (rhytidectomy). In: Myers EN, editor. Operate otolaryngology: head and neck surgery. Philadelphia: Saunders; 2003. p. 846 66.
31. Karacaoğlan N, Akbaş H. Effect of parenteral pentoxifylline and topical nitroglycerin on skin flap survival. Otolaryngol Head Neck Surg 1999;120(2):272–4.

Recognizing and Managing Complications in Laser Resurfacing, Chemical Peels, and Dermabrasion

Mark M. Hamilton, MD*, Richard Kao, MD

KEYWORDS

- Laser resurfacing • Chemical peel • Dermabrasion • Infection • Hypopigmentation • Scarring
- Hyperpigmentation • Complications

KEY POINTS

- Laser resurfacing, chemical peels, and dermabrasion are all associated with overlapping complications including infection, hypopigmentation, hyperpigmentation, and scarring. In general, more aggressive treatments are associated with a higher rate of complications.
- Fractional laser resurfacing techniques offer treatments with a lower overall rate of complications including almost negligible risk hypopigmentation. The downside to these treatments is that multiple treatments are required to achieve similar results.
- A thorough understanding of the Glogau scale and the Fitzpatrick scale will help to optimize treatment to the patient while minimizing the risk of complications.

Skin resurfacing techniques are some of the most satisfying procedures performed by facial plastic surgeons and other cosmetic providers. Lasers, chemical peels, and dermabrasion – as the primary treatment or as an adjunct to surgical management – are valuable tools in the arsenal of skin rejuvenation. These techniques have proven effective in effacing wrinkles, removing skin discolorations, and softening scars. Although powerful tools, these modalities can produce potentially unfavorable results. This article will focus on potential complications from all of these techniques. It is the authors' hope that knowledge of these adverse effects will first and foremost help readers avoid these complications, but just as important promptly recognize them when they do occur and provide definitive treatment thereafter.

Although there is some variance, there is a great deal of overlap of the types of complications and their frequency among all 3 methods. These include initial concerns of patient safety such as ocular injury or fire. Immediate postoperative concerns are mostly infectious and most commonly viral. Later complications include pigmentary issues and scarring. The authors will cover these in sequential order.

PATIENT EVALUATION

An important part of avoiding complications is patient evaluation. The first part of this is determining the level of photodamage or scarring to be treated. The Glogau scale is an excellent tool to categorize the severity (**Fig. 1**). In general, those patients with higher scores require more aggressive treatments that typically have a higher risk of complications.

Department of Otolaryngology-Head and Neck Surgery, Indiana University School of Medicine, 340 West 10 th Street, Fairbanks Hall, Suite 6200, Indianapolis, IN 46202-3082, USA
* Corresponding author. Hamilton Facial Plastic Surgery, 533 East County Line Road, suite #104, Greenwood, IN 46143.
E-mail address: mmckhamilton@gmail.com

Facial Plast Surg Clin N Am 28 (2020) 493–501
https://doi.org/10.1016/j.fsc.2020.06.008

THE GLOGAU SCALE

SKIN TYPE	CLASSIFICATION	AGE	SKIN CHARACTERISTICS
TYPE I	Mild	28–35	No Wrinkles Early photo aging: mild pigment changes, no keratosis, minimal wrinkles, minimal or no makeup
TYPE II	Moderate	35–50	Wrinkles in motion Early to moderate photo aging: early brown spots visible, keratosis palpable but not visible, parallel smile lines begin to appear, wears more foundation
TYPE III	Advanced	50-65	Wrinkles at Rest Advanced photo aging: obvious discoloration, visible capillaries, visible keratosis, wears heavier makeup
TYPE IV	Severe	60 & Up	Only Wrinkles Severe photo aging: yellow/grey skin color, prior skin malignancies, wrinkles throughout - no normal skin, cannot wear make-up because it cracks and cakes

Fig. 1. Glogau scale.

Those patients who have lower scores can receive less aggressive treatments and thus decrease the likelihood of complications.

The other important guideline is the Fitzpatrick scale (**Fig. 2**). In general, those patients with lower scores carry a lower risk of postprocedure pigmentary issues and scarring and are more likely to tolerate more aggressive forms of treatment. The opposite is true for higher scores. Fortunately, patients with higher Fitzpatrick scores rarely have higher Glogau scores and thus rarely need the more aggressive methods.

If there is any doubt about how a patient may tolerate a treatment, a test patch can be performed in a less obvious area. The practitioner can follow the healing process and note the resulting complications. This can be used to guide the choice of method for the definitive treatment.

PERIOCULAR INJURY

Injury to the orbit can be catastrophic, and its avoidance is a top concern. Corneal injuries are most commonly associated with CO_2 and Erbium lasers.[1,2] Extensive laser safety precautions must be taken when using any laser resurfacing methods. For Erbium and CO_2 laser around the eye, intraocular metal shields are essential. For other lasers or procedures that are done away from the eyes, laser-proof glasses specific to the laser type may be appropriate. It is important to confirm the safety glasses are specific for the wavelength of the laser being utilized. In addition, all personnel in the laser suite must be also wear eye protection during the laser procedure. Obviously, the practitioner performing the procedure must be trained in proper use of the device, but also important is that the nursing staff is trained properly and certified for laser use.

Ocular injury is also a concern with chemical peel procedures. It is always important to have a dry cotton-tip applicator available while peeling around the eyes. Tears should be immediately dried to avoid wicking of the peel agent into the eyes. In addition, balanced saline solution should be readily available to irrigate out the eye should an injury occur. For deep chemical peels involving phenol, mineral oil should be available. This is used to irrigate the eye (instead of saline) if phenol accidently encounters the eye tissues. Because eyelid skin is extremely thin and easily torn, dermabrasion to the eyelid area should be approached with extreme caution. Intraocular metal shields are

THE FITZPATRICK SCALE

SKIN TYPE	APPEARANCE	DETAILS
TYPE I	Pale to very fair skin Red or blond hair Light colored eyes May have freckles	Always burn Never tans High risk of skin cancer and vascular damage
TYPE II	Fair skin Light eyes Light hair	Burns easily Rarely tans High risk of skin cancer and vascular damage
TYPE III	Fair skin Medium to dark hair Eye color may vary	Sometimes burns Tans gradually Risk of hyper/hypopigmentation Moderate risk of skin cancer and vascular damage
TYPE IV	Light brown to tanned skin Dark hair and eyes	Burns easily Rarely tans High risk of skin cancer and vascular damage
TYPE V	Dark skin Dark eyes Dark hair	Skin darkens but never burns High risk of hyper/hypopigmentation Scars easily Moderate risk of vascular damage
TYPE VI	Very dark skin Dark eyes Dark hair	Tans easily but never burns Very high risk of hyper/hypopigmenation High risk of scarring Moderate risk of vascular damage Low risk of aging and skin damage from sun exsposure

Fig. 2. Fitzpatrick scale.

required if dermabrasion is done anywhere near the eye area.

It is important to note that the risk of ectropion is present with laser and chemexfoliation. The incidence of ectropion is 0.4% with laser resurfacing of the lower eyelid.[3] This can occur as a result of healing contracture but is usually caused by excessive resurfacing of the thin and highly contractile skin of the lower eyelids.[4] When lid retraction does appear after treatment, conservative treatment with massage and eye protection should be done first. In minor cases, the lid position is restored once the contraction releases, and can by aided by triamcinolone injections. In severe cases, lid tightening procedures may be required if there is no improvement after a period of 3 to 6 months.

Risk factors include previous blepharoplasty, concurrent surgeries, and laxity of the lower lid. Proper preoperative evaluation should include lid laxity test and snap test. Poor eyelid tone preoperatively may necessitate lower lid tightening or tarsal strip procedure prior to resurfacing. Treatment of the middle lamella and excessive collagen contraction can also contribute to development of ectropion.[5]

LASER FIRE

This complication is unique to lasers and fortunately a rare one. Fire and explosion can occur whenever a laser beam is directed at a flammable object. This can include dry sponges and drapes, hair products, oxygen, alcohol-based preparations, and endotracheal tubes. All towels and sponges should be wet, and the endotracheal tube should be covered with wet gauze or towels. A large basin of water and a fire extinguisher should be immediately available if a fire does occur.

INFECTION

Infections and their sequelae can be serious complications after resurfacing. Fortunately, they are generally treatable and should be identified early to facilitate prompt management. This can help to prevent scarring, delayed wound healing, propagation of infection, and colonization of opportunistic pathogens.

Viral

Postresurfacing viral infections present with the small superficial lesions, often with the presence of vesicles and pustules. These can have associated burning, paresthesia, and drainage. Herpes simplex virus (HSV) is the most common infection observed with all skin resurfacing techniques. Herpetic lesions present with disproportionately painful vesicular eruptions, often within a dermatome distribution.

Pretreatment regimens vary among practitioners. For instance, some advocate for prophylactic treatment for each patient regardless of history of HSV outbreak, as most patients contain this latent virus despite the absence of symptoms.[6] Others challenge this in the use of fractional CO_2 and erbium doped laser, as these methods produce a reported 1.1% to 1.7% incidence of HSV outbreak. These studies thus concluded that antiviral prophylaxis for all patients is likely unnecessary.[7,8] Some recommend that antiviral prophylaxis be given only in those having history of HSV outbreak.[9] Prophylactic treatment is recommended for all medium and deep chemical peels, dermabrasion, and full-field laser resurfacing procedures that involve the perioral area.

Prophylactic postresurfacing treatment should continue for 1 to 2 weeks (or until skin exfoliation is complete and the skin barrier is restored) for those with prior history of herpesvirus infections. The authors' regimen for full field resurfacing is typically Valacyclovir 500 mg twice daily for 2 weeks starting 3 days before for patients with a history of herpetic outbreaks and the day before for all other patients.

If lesions are detected, postresurfacing herpetic infections should be aggressively treated with oral and topical antiviral medications due to the risk of tissue necrosis from the resulting vasculitis. In our patients, the oral dose is doubled (valacyclovir 1 g twice daily) at the first sign of infection. In severe cases, scarring may develop and can be treated with injectable steroids or scar revision.

Bacterial

Postresurfacing bacterial infections present with facial swelling, erythema, and discharge. They commonly occur 2 to 10 days after resurfacing.[10] The most common offending bacterial organisms include *Staphylococcus, Pseudomonas, Klebsiella,* and *Enterobacter.*[11] Thick yellow crusting is observed with *S aureus,* whereas a characteristic odor is observed with *Pseudomonas.*

The rate of incidence is between 0.5% and 4.5%.[12] Antibiotic prophylaxis is understandably controversial, given the risk of developing drug-resistant bacteria.[13] In fact, use of antibiotics showed no reduction in infection rate in a retrospective study using CO_2 laser.[14] Most bacterial infections develop because of insufficient removal of debris during the exfoliation process. Detailed instructions and close patient follow-up are critical to prevention and early treatment, especially with full-field laser resurfacing treatments and medium or deep chemical peels. These patients are either seen daily during the initial healing period or at least contacted by phone to closely monitor their progress.

If a bacterial infection is observed, oral antibiotic therapy should be initiated. Antibiotics should cover *S aureus* and *Pseudomonas* species and may be combined with concurrent antiviral therapy. Just as important is topical treatment. Starting patients on a regimen using 0.25% acetic acid soaks (formula = 1 quart: 3 Tbsp white vinegar + 1 quart lukewarm water) will help remove excess debris and most effectively treat the infection.

Fungal

Fungal infections will typically present with irregular patches of erythema and exudates or reticular white patches. Candida albicans is the most common fungal infection after resurfacing treatments. Although rare, fungal infections are associated with use of topical antibiotics, diabetes, immunosuppression, and angular cheilitis.[15]

The rate of incidence is between 0% and 1.2% of patients.[9,16] When observed, these infections can typically be treated with a topical antifungal such as ketoconazole as well as an oral agent like fluconazole. Like bacterial infections, poor debridement and cleaning may play a role. Starting acetic acid wash can reverse this and treat the infection. It has been suggested that pretreatment antifungal agents may be appropriate in patients with frequent vaginal yeast infections.[17]

HYPERPIGMENTATION

Hyperpigmentation is the most common complication of skin resurfacing. It is the product of hypermelanosis of the skin after skin resurfacing.[18] It is often attributed to unintentional and unprotected sun exposure, which exacerbates the hyperpigmentation process.[19]

Hyperpigmentation will typically present 3 to 4 weeks after resurfacing treatment, and in most cases will self-resolve over the span of weeks to months. However, this condition may persist up to 6 to 9 months, causing a potentially great amount of distress to patients.

Generally, the risk of hyperpigmentation increases with darker skin types.[20] The most common scale used to describe skin pigmentation is the Fitzpatrick skin type scale (see **Fig. 2**). Specifically, those patients exhibiting Fitzpatrick skin types IV through VI are at the highest risk of hyperpigmentation. It is thought that higher heat, frequency, and duration of resurfacing causes increased pigmentation. Treatment selection should be individualized to the patient's skin type to prevent or at least minimize the risk of hyperpigmentation.

Hyperpigmentation occurs in 30% of all patients after CO_2 laser resurfacing and nearly 100% of dark-skinned patients.[16] It can occur in those with lighter skin types I, II, and III also.[15] A review of 8 studies revealed that hyperpigmentation in fractional erbium-doped laser ranges widely between 1% to 32% of patients.[12] Most studies, however, have shown fractional laser devices to have significantly lower rates of hyperpigmentation compare with full-field laser devices (**Fig. 3**).

Given the relatively high incidence of hyperpigmentation, counseling and implementation of a pretreatment topical regimen may be considered. Patients are advised to apply sunscreen with 15+ SPF for at least 4 weeks prior to resurfacing and to continue use after treatment to maintain results.[21] In Fitzpatrick IV through VI skin types, prophylactic pretreatment of topical hydroquinone up to 4 weeks before resurfacing may be helpful with preventing hyperpigmentation. Sun avoidance for several weeks before and after is critical. In general, the authors advise patients to avoid the sun after resurfacing procedures until any pink discoloration has completely faded.

When delayed-onset hyperpigmentation is observed, treatment must include use of broad-spectrum sunscreen, and will typically include hydroquinone and/or light glycolic acid peels.[21] In fact, use of 4% hydroquinone has been shown to decrease hyperpigmentation from 21% to 6%.[22] Application should be performed on the affected

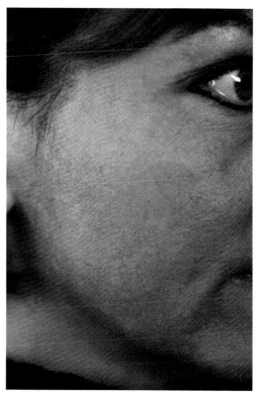

Fig. 3. Hyperpigmentation after full face CO_2 laser resurfacing.

areas and surrounding skin to help with skin tone blending. Other bleaching agents such as kojic acid and azelaic acid also may be used, especially if long-term treatment is required.

HYPOPIGMENTATION

The development of hypopigmentation after skin resurfacing is caused by irreversible damage of the melanocytes, thereby disrupting melanogenesis. First, it is important to differentiate between hypopigmentation and pseudohypopigmentation. Pseudohypopigmentation occurs when sun-damaged skin, which is darker than normal for the patient, becomes appropriately lighter and consistent with normal pigmentation after treatment.[22] Therefore, the patient receiving resurfacing should be counseled in preoperative discussions that lines of demarcation can be expected between areas of treatment. For instance, if only the face is treated, there is a high likelihood of delineation between the lightened face and the darker, untreated sun-damaged neck skin.

In general, true hypopigmentation as a complication of resurfacing is observed up to 6 to 12 months after the treatment.[21] The risk of hypopigmentation increases when the resurfacing depth penetrates too deeply into the reticular dermis,[19] and also increases with the amount of thermal injury to the treated areas.[21] It is caused by irreversible damage of the melanocytes, which exist at the papillary-reticular dermal junction. Hypopigmentation tends to occur in areas of skin that have received high-intensity resurfacing, and also in areas that have received multiple resurfacing modalities of resurfacing.[15] Hypopigmentation is most noticeable in the presence of hyperpigmentation or melanosis, which is most often exhibited by Asian and Hispanic patients.[19]

The risk of hypopigmentation for all resurfacing techniques is reported to be as high as 8%.[9] Of note, the risk decreases significantly with fractional laser device use versus older full-field ablative lasers.

Unfortunately, this unsightly complication may be irreversible in some cases. In these instances, the darker skin surrounding the depigmented areas is treated with chemical peels to minimize the stark demarcations. This allows for smoother blending of the depigmented areas into the now paler native skin.[23] Selective treatment of the entire face can also be performed to further decrease the contrast between multiple areas of depigmentation and untreated skin. This is performed using glycolic acid peels and light trichloroacetic acid peels.[21] In addition, fractionated 1550 nm erbium-doped laser combined with topical bimatoprost and tretinoin or pimecrolimus has been used to treat hypopigmentation.[24]

It is important to discuss the potential for hypopigmentation for patients before resurfacing. Patients should be selected for treatments based on their Fitzpatrick type. In general, deep chemical peels, full-field laser resurfacing and aggressive dermabrasion treatments are reserved for those with lighter skin types (I, II, and occasionally III). Fractional laser treatments and light chemical peels can be done for darker skin types but should be approached with caution.

In addition, full-face treatments should be the default when treatments carry the risks of hypopigmentation to avoid lines of demarcation on the face. This allows the line of demarcation between the line of treatment of the face and the untreated neck to be partially hidden under the mandible. Even so, feathering should be performed to avoid a well-defined line of demarcation. This same principle of feathering should be employed if regional treatments are attempted (**Fig. 4**).

PROLONGED ERYTHEMA

Postresurfacing erythema, although cosmetically displeasing to patients, is a part of normal healing that is expected to occur after resurfacing. A measured amount of inflammation will occur after any resurfacing technique, as portions of the epidermis and papillary and reticular dermis are ablated. It is critical to understand the type of resurfacing technique to determine whether the postoperative erythema is within the expected time frame. For instance, superficial chemical peels will typically cause erythema of 3 to 5 days, whereas medium depth peels will cause 15 to 30 days of erythema. With deep chemical peels, some erythema may be expected for the first 2 to 3 months.[25] A similar time frame would

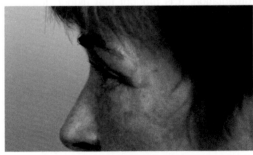

Fig. 4. Periocular hypopigmentation caused by regional CO_2 laser resurfacing.

be expected for full-field laser resurfacing procedures.

Laser resurfacing alone demonstrates a wide variability in postoperative erythema. For instance, lasers such as ablative CO_2 and Er:YAG have been shown to produce postoperative erythema of at least 3.6 and 4.5 weeks respectively,[26] but in some cases will last up to 2 to 4 months in the authors' experience. With fractional CO_2 laser treatments of the face, only 1% of patients have erythema longer than 4 days.[8]

Persistent erythema can also occur from allergic or irritant contact dermatitis, exacerbation of a pre-existing skin condition, or superficial infections. A multitude of topical creams, ointments, toners, and cleansers may contribute to contact dermatitis in the postoperative period. If an offending agent is identified, this should be immediately discontinued.[27] Moreover, antimicrobial topical ointments such as bacitracin, neomycin, and polymyxin are discouraged because of increased risk of dermatitis and so-called paraffinomas.[28,29] Patients should be instructed to avoid use of these antimicrobial ointments.

Prolonged erythema can be treated using multiple methodologies. Topical treatments include hydrocortisone 1% cream, hydrocortisone 2.5% cream, hydrocortisone valerate 0.2% cream,[21] and topical ascorbic acid after re-epithelialization.[10] Response is expected within 2 to 3 weeks.[25] These topical ointments are applied after re-epithelialization, typically occurring after 4 to 7 days, to avoid disruption of wound healing. The use of steroid creams prior to re-epithelialization has been associated with increased infection rates.[30] However, use of intense pulsed Er:YAG laser has been used to remove erythema and hyperpigmentation after CO_2 laser resurfacing of the periorbital area[31] (**Fig. 5**).

Importantly, prolonged intense redness may indicate prolonged fibroplasia, which can lead to skin thickening and scarring. Development of hypertrophic scarring after erythema is often observed in the perioral areas.[32]

SCARRING

Hypertrophic scars are the most devastating complication of resurfacing.[4,33] As stated in the previous section, scarring may be preceded by abnormal erythema or induration. Post-treatment scarring will occur if the depth of resurfacing penetrates too deeply into the reticular dermis, and the skin is unable to heal in a normal fashion.[34] With respect to laser resurfacing, it is thought to be caused by high energy density, inadvertent pulse stacking, and overly aggressive treatment with the laser.[35] Preoperative assessment should include evaluation of personal or family history of autoimmune diseases. Disorders such as vitiligo and psoriasis have been documented to cause dermatoses or keratoacanthomas. This so-called Koebnerization process has been described in laser resurfacing.[36]

Scarring tends to occur 2 to 4 weeks postoperatively.[12] It is observed in 2% to 4% of all laser resurfacing cases.[35] Although some cases of hypertrophic scarring after fractional CO_2 laser use have been described,[4,10,34] the reported risk is much lower. The largest published case series of over 2000 subjects reported no incidence of hypertrophic scar after use of a fractional CO_2 laser.[10]

Within the face, hypertrophic scarring is found most often in the upper lip, neck, periorbital area, and mandible areas. The neck and chest, which have much thinner skin, tend to be more susceptible to scarring than the face.[34]

A variety of treatments may be used to treat hypertrophic scarring. These includes topical steroids, intralesional steroid injection, intralesional 5-fluorouracil injection, occlusive dressings, pulsed dye laser, repeat light fractional resurfacing, or broadband light therapy.[22] With less severe scars characterized by small fibrotic bands, patients may benefit from massaging the area 3 to 4 times per day with silicone-based scar fading creams. Also helpful is silicone sheeting. Firmer, more prominent scars should be treated with intralesional steroid injection using Kenalog K-10 suspension. The steroid injection should be limited to the scar band area only, as injection in excess can lead to atrophy of the subcutaneous fat and produce an undesired depression. Injection should be performed at 3- to 6-week intervals and can be titrated to higher concentrations as needed.

Regimens have been described using intralesional triamcinolone 10 mg/mL or 5-fluorouracil along with pulsed dye laser treatment for the

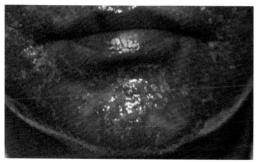

Fig. 5. Herpetic outbreak after perioral laser resurfacing.

resolution of hypertrophic scars.[10,17] These treatments contribute to decreasing collagen production, reducing extracellular matrix deposition and modulating growth factors involved with wound healing.[37] Scars refractory to the treatments already mentioned may ultimately require surgical scar revision.

MILIA

Milia are superficial inclusion cysts limited within the epidermis during the re-epithelialization process. Milia are considered common side effects, occurring as often as 50% of the time in patients within 4 weeks after dermabrasion,[38] and thus they are not considered a true complication. Although most milia self-resolve, the larger ones can be uncapped with an 18-gauge needle or pinpoint electrodessication for quick resolution. Post-treatment topical 0.05% retinol ointment has also been shown to be effective in reducing milia incidence.[39]

OTHER CONSIDERATIONS

Acne treatment must be approached carefully, as the recently re-epithelialized skin is more sensitive after resurfacing.

Systemic toxicity may be observed with chemical peels as salicylate and phenol toxicity. It is not typically observed after peeling of small surface areas, such as facial skin.[40] High systemic absorption of salicylic acid, which is commonly used in superficial peels or Jessner solution, presents with nausea and vomiting, flushing, tinnitus, tachypnea, and convulsions or comas in more severe cases. In mild-to-moderate cases, treatment includes intravenous (IV) fluid hydration, correction of metabolic acidosis, and serial serum levels. Patients presenting with altered mental status indicate a more severe toxicity and would necessitate a head computed tomography (CT) scan to rule out cerebral edema.

Phenol is a common ingredient found in chemical peels such as Baker-Gordon and Hetter solution. The most important risk with these peels is cardiac arrhythmias and the risk of sudden death.[41] Phenol is also toxic to the liver and kidneys. To avoid toxicity, treatments should be staged, allowing 15 minutes between application of facial subunits. Patients should also be hydrated in advance and during the procedure with IV fluids. Additionally, patients should receive continuous cardiac monitoring and supplemental oxygen. Toxic levels are typically between 50 to 500 mg/kg.

SUMMARY

Complications from resurfacing procedures will occur even with the most careful of preparation and execution. Thorough physician knowledge of these possible adverse effects will go a long way toward decreasing the potential and improving recognition and prompt and appropriate treatment when they do arise. The prepared physician will be able to minimize the downside when these complications occur and improve the overall result and patient experience.

DISCLOSURE

M.M. Hamilton: Speakers bureau, Allergan; R. Kao: Nothing to disclose.

REFERENCES

1. Barkana Y, Belkin M. Laser eye injuries. Surv Ophthalmol 2000;44:459–78.
2. Lund DJ, Landers MB, Bresnick GH, et al. Ocular hazards of the Q-switched erbium laser. Invest Ophthalmol 1970;9:463–70.
3. Apfelberg DB. Summary of the 1997 ASAPS/ASPRS Laser Task Force survey on laser resurfacing and laser blepharoplasty. American Society for Aesthetic Plastic Surgery. American Society of Plastic and Reconstructive Surgeons. Plast Reconstr Surg 1998;101:511–8.
4. Fife DJ, Fitzpatrick RE, Zachary CB. Complications of fractional CO2 laser resurfacing: four cases. Lasers Surg Med 2009;41:179–84.
5. Alster TS, Khoury RR. Treatment of laser complications. Facial Plast Surg 2009;25:316–23.
6. Spruance SL. The natural history of recurrent oral-facial herpes simplex virus infection. Semin Dermatol 1992;11:200–6.
7. Graber EM, Tanzi EL, Alster TS. Side effects and complications of fractional laser photothermolysis: experience with 961 treatments. Dermatol Surg 2008;34:301–5 [discussion: 5-7].
8. Campbell TM, Goldman MP. Adverse events of fractionated carbon dioxide laser: review of 373 treatments. Dermatol Surg 2010;36:1645–50.
9. Shamsaldeen O, Peterson JD, Goldman MP. The adverse events of deep fractional CO(2): a retrospective study of 490 treatments in 374 patients. Lasers Surg Med 2011;43:453–6.
10. Hunzeker CM, Weiss ET, Geronemus RG. Fractionated CO2 laser resurfacing: our experience with more than 2000 treatments. Aesthet Surg J 2009; 29:317–22.
11. Ramsdell WM. Fractional CO2 Laser Resurfacing Complications. Semin Plast Surg 2012;26:137–40.

12. Metelitsa AI, Alster TS. Fractionated laser skin resurfacing treatment complications: a review. Dermatol Surg 2010;36:299–306.

13. Alster TS. Cutaneous resurfacing with CO2 and erbium: YAG lasers: preoperative, intraoperative, and postoperative considerations. Plast Reconstr Surg 1999;103:619–32 [discussion: 33–4].

14. Walia S, Alster TS. Cutaneous CO2 laser resurfacing infection rate with and without prophylactic antibiotics. Dermatol Surg 1999;25:857–61.

15. Alster TS, Lupton JR. Treatment of complications of laser skin resurfacing. Arch Facial Plast Surg 2000; 2:279–84.

16. Weinstein C, Pozner JN, Ramirez OM. Complications of carbon dioxide laser resurfacing and their prevention. Aesthet Surg J 1997;17:216–25.

17. Fitzpatrick RE, Williams B, Goldman MP. Preoperative anesthesia and postoperative considerations in laser resurfacing. Semin Cutan Med Surg 1996;15: 170–6.

18. Oram Y, Akkaya AD. Refractory postinflammatory hyperpigmentation treated fractional CO2 laser. J Clin Aesthet Dermatol 2014;7:42–4.

19. Apfelberg DB. Side effects, sequelae, and complications of carbon dioxide resurfacing. Aesthet Surg J 1997;17:365–72.

20. Monheit GD. Chemical peels. Skin Ther Lett 2004;9: 6–11.

21. Alster TS, Lupton JR. Prevention and treatment of side effects and complications of cutaneous laser resurfacing. Plast Reconstr Surg 2002;109:308–16 [discussion: 17–8].

22. Schwartz RJ, Burns AJ, Rohrich RJ, et al. Long-term assessment of CO2 facial laser resurfacing: aesthetic results and complications. Plast Reconstr Surg 1999;103:592–601.

23. McBurney EI. Side effects and complications of laser therapy. Dermatol Clin 2002;20:165–76.

24. Massaki AB, Fabi SG, Fitzpatrick R. Repigmentation of hypopigmented scars using an erbium-doped 1,550-nm fractionated laser and topical bimatoprost. Dermatol Surg 2012;38:995–1001.

25. Langsdon PR, Shires CB. Chemical face peeling. Facial Plast Surg 2012;28:116–25.

26. Tanzi EL, Alster TS. Single-pass carbon dioxide versus multiple-pass Er:YAG laser skin resurfacing: a comparison of postoperative wound healing and side-effect rates. Dermatol Surg 2003;29:80–4.

27. Lowe NJ, Lask G, Griffin ME. Laser skin resurfacing. Pre- and posttreatment guidelines. Dermatol Surg 1995;21:1017–9.

28. Fisher AA. Topical medicaments which are common sensitizers. Ann Allergy 1982;49:97–100.

29. Fisher AA. Lasers and allergic contact dermatitis to topical antibiotics, with particular reference to bacitracin. Cutis 1996;58:252–4.

30. Ortiz AE, Tingey C, Yu YE, et al. Topical steroids implicated in postoperative infection following ablative laser resurfacing. Lasers Surg Med 2012;44: 1–3.

31. Kontoes PP, Vlachos SP, Marayiannis KV. Intense pulsed light for the treatment of lentigines in LEOPARD syndrome. Br J Plast Surg 2003;56:607–10.

32. Brody HJ. Complications of chemical peeling. J Dermatol Surg Oncol 1989;15:1010–9.

33. Ross EV, Grossman MC, Duke D, et al. Long-term results after CO2 laser skin resurfacing: a comparison of scanned and pulsed systems. J Am Acad Dermatol 1997;37:709–18.

34. Avram MM, Tope WD, Yu T, et al. Hypertrophic scarring of the neck following ablative fractional carbon dioxide laser resurfacing. Lasers Surg Med 2009; 41:185–8.

35. Riggs K, Keller M, Humphreys TR. Ablative laser resurfacing: high-energy pulsed carbon dioxide and erbium:yttrium-aluminum-garnet. Clin Dermatol 2007;25:462–73.

36. Mamelak AJ, Goldberg LH, Marquez D, et al. Eruptive keratoacanthomas on the legs after fractional photothermolysis: report of two cases. Dermatol Surg 2009;35:513–8.

37. Cohen JL, Ross EV. Combined fractional ablative and nonablative laser resurfacing treatment: a split-face comparative study. J Drugs Dermatol 2013;12:175–8.

38. Yarborough JM, Beeson WH. Aesthetic surgery of the aging face. In: Beeson WH, editor. Aesthetic surgery of the aging face. Mosby; 1986. p. 142–58.

39. Mandy SH. Tretinoin in the preoperative and postoperative management of dermabrasion. J Am Acad Dermatol 1986;15:878–9, 88-89.

40. Landau M. Chemical peels. Clin Dermatol 2008;26: 200–8.

41. Landau M. Cardiac complications in deep chemical peels. Dermatol Surg 2007;33:190–3 [discussion: 3].

Life in an Academic Practice Versus a Solo Private Practice: How Different Are They?

Fred G. Fedok, MD[a],*, Jessyka G. Lighthall, MD[b], Jordan Rihani, MD[c]

KEYWORDS

- Facial plastic surgery • Academic practice • Private practice • Human resources • Schedule
- Life balance

KEY POINTS

- There are many similarities and differences in the practices of academic and private practice facial plastic surgeons.
- Private practice offers more autonomy than academic practice. With autonomy there is more individual responsibility and risk.
- Academic practice offers more opportunities for research and organizational leadership growth than private practice.
- Human resource management is a central concern for surgeons in both academic and private practice settings.

INTRODUCTION
Fred G. Fedok

To be transparent, I have been largely responsible for the assembly of this panel of dedicated facial plastic surgeons who have been kind to share their views and experiences. It was proposed that the format of this article would be based on their answers to a series of questions about their varied practice settings. These questions were created after requesting that each individual author submit questions about what they thought would probe pertinent issues and differences in their practices. After receiving everyone's questions they were then asked to rank the compiled list of questions according to what they felt to be pertinent to their individual practices and reveal insights that might be of help to others. Those 6 questions that were ranked the highest form the basis of the article.

The aim of this "study" and article is to communicate similarities and differences in the lives of those practicing in "Academic" versus "Private" practice settings. None of the authors saw the other panel members' answers until they had been incorporated into one document. Meanwhile I have related my own personal experiences while trying to avoid, as much as possible, influence by seeing the answers of the other authors.

CURRENT PRACTICE ENVIRONMENT
Jessyka G. Lighthall

I work in an academic practice with a university-based functional and reconstructive clinic in the general Otolaryngology and Pediatric Surgery clinical suite with 6 physician's assistants and university-based operative block time 5 sessions per month. In addition, I travel to an outpatient

All authors equally contributed.
[a] Department of Surgery, University of South Alabama Mobile, Fedok Plastic Surgery, 113 East Fern Avenue, Foley, AL 36535, USA; [b] Facial Plastic & Reconstructive Surgery, Department of Otolaryngology–Head & Neck Surgery, Penn State College of Medicine, 500 University Drive H-091, Hershey, PA 17033, USA; [c] Facial Plastic Surgery Institute, Southlake, TX 76092, USA
* Corresponding author.
E-mail address: drfredfedok@me.com

Facial Plast Surg Clin N Am 28 (2020) 503–514
https://doi.org/10.1016/j.fsc.2020.07.001
1064-7406/20/© 2020 Elsevier Inc. All rights reserved.

surgery center where I perform cosmetic facial procedures, as well as to an off-site cosmetic center to evaluate patients and perform minimally invasive procedures. Several clinic sessions per month I run a multidisciplinary Facial Nerve Disorders Clinic approximately 5 minutes from the university and have 1 academic day per week.

Jordan Rihani

I am in my fourth year of practice as a solo practitioner. I have 2 locations and employ 3 full-time and 1 part-time administrative/clinical staff. My practice is mainly cosmetic surgical procedures, followed by injectables and Mohs reconstructive procedures.

I am in an office-sharing arrangement with 2 plastic surgeons with a simple rent payment arrangement (**Fig. 1**). I have my own staff and separate finances. They are busy practitioners that have been in practice for more than 15 years and focus on breast and body work, referring any aging face patients to me. I do have an operating room in one of my offices where I perform some of my cosmetic procedures.

Fred G. Fedok

Currently I am in a solo private practice in Foley, Alabama-Fedok Plastic Surgery. The practice is focused on rejuvenation of the aging face and related issues and incorporates most of the surgical, minimally invasive, and nonsurgical aspects of the discipline. We are also engaged in the wider discipline of facial plastic surgery, including rhinoplasty, hair transplantation, laser and light procedures, care of cutaneous malignancies, and reconstructive procedures. By far, however, the largest clinical volume is in the area of patients seeking care for aging face concerns.

My current office configuration includes a waiting room, a front office, a back-staff office, a manger-coordinator office, 2 examination-consultation rooms, my professional office/consultation office, a dedicated laser and light procedure suite, and a large procedure-operating suite (**Figs. 2–5**). I am situated across the street from a regional medical center, so that my more involved procedures and general anesthesia cases are performed there. We use the Modernizing Medicine electronic medical record so there is no need for a medical record room. There are 5 full-time and 2 part-time employees.

For those who do not know me, I must add that I spent approximately 25 years in academic practice and now have spent the past 5 years in private practice. The experience has been nothing short of enlightening in noting the differences in practicing within a large university practice versus a solo private practice.

QUESTION 1. ON A DAY-TO-DAY BASIS, WHAT ARE YOUR TOP 3 CHALLENGES?
Jessyka G. Lighthall

Facial plastic surgery is a unique practice environment with specific subspecialty requirements, such as higher staffing needs, increased marketing costs, and potentially significant cosmetic equipment costs (eg, lasers); fulfilling these needs is what I struggle with on a daily basis.

The academic environment poses several challenges to the following:

1. *Scheduling:* Scheduling of clinics are a challenge primarily due to the complexity of having 3 separate outpatient clinic sites managed by different scheduling staff. Schedulers manage multiple specialties as well as the multidisciplinary clinics and work off of a predetermined template with minimal flexibility. Although protocols are provided, the schedulers have no knowledge of the individual physician or practice nuances. Physicians must be consistently

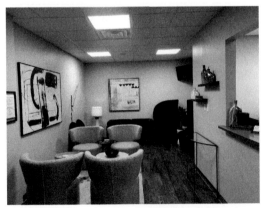

Fig. 1. Rihani waiting room/reception area, Fort Worth location facial plastic surgery.

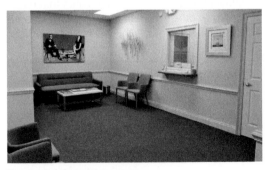

Fig. 2. Fedok waiting room.

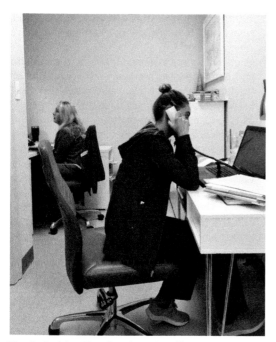

Fig. 3. Fedok office for clinical staff.

reviewing their clinic schedules to ensure patient care is optimized and clinical efficiency is maintained.

2. *Preauthorization process:* The second challenge in my practice is obtaining timely preauthorizations for services (clinic-based and operative procedures). This includes chemodenervation for sialorrhea or synkinesis and all functional or reconstructive operative cases. This a time-consuming process for staff who have multiple other duties within their job descriptions (eg, scheduling of operating room [OR] cases for multiple providers). From a physician viewpoint, this significantly affects our ability to care for patients if authorizations are not obtained in a timely fashion before

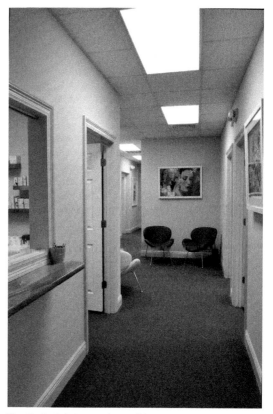

Fig. 5. Fedok intrasuite waiting area.

surgery, with procedures being canceled or postponed at the last minute. Recurrent authorization issues can decrease physician job satisfaction and the satisfaction of staff involved. In addition, this may impact overall patient satisfaction scores for the provider and institution, as patients often wait months for their surgery, have taken time off work, and arranged for childcare and assistance at home. As we know, in the current environment, patient satisfaction ratings can have a significant impact on a practice. Many aspects of the patient experience, from ease with scheduling, preauthorizations, waiting time to surgery, resident team, ability to reach someone with questions, clinic delays, or parking, are unrelated to the physician's clinical acumen or surgical skill but intimately entwined to the overall patient experience. To circumvent issues in obtaining authorizations that delay patient care, we created a preauthorization position dedicated solely to obtaining authorizations.

3. *Balance:* Finally, in an academic setting, there is a fine balance between providing high-

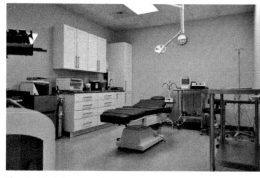

Fig. 4. Fedok procedure room.

quality patient care, educating learners, performing and publishing research, and completing required administrative work. The top challenge for me is the balance of maintaining a productive and rewarding clinical practice while allowing time for other academic requirements and interests and maintaining the healthy family environment.

These challenges are important to address, as burnout among plastic surgeons specifically has been attributed to long work hours and frequent calls, emotional exhaustion, poor to fair health of the physician, lack of autonomy and control over practice environment, and imbalance between career and family.[1]

Jordan Rihani

1. *Patient care:* Despite the challenges of running your own business, the main challenge of a medical practice is, and should be, delivering high-quality patient care and surgical outcomes. If your outcomes are not your primary concern, then other issues will most certainly arise, such as lack of patient retention and dealing with negative press/reviews.Patient care does not stop when surgery is over. On the contrary, that is when it begins. This entails following up with patients regularly with scheduled clinic visits and phone calls. This maintains open communication lines, helps with recognition of issues, and facilitates solutions. I believe in maintaining these communication channels with patients as much as possible to avoid them feeling isolated or helpless. This means that if a patient wants to talk to me, it's not hard for them to get me directly. I also e-mail semi-annual, anonymous surveys to my patients to monitor how we are doing as a practice. Patients all have questions that, when not answered appropriately, leave them feeling confused and frustrated.
2. *Marketing and brand management:* There are limitless opportunities to market your practice, whether magazine and print advertisements, "pay per click" Internet advertising, Web site development, search engine optimization, or local community event sponsorships. The question is "which opportunities provide the best return on investment of my time and money?" Even "free advertising" like Instagram or Facebook can actually be quite expensive from a time perspective (**Figs. 6** and **7**). Thorough understanding of your budget as well your target population is the key to successful, efficient marketing. In a solo practice I have 100% control over my advertising budget and what I want to be investing my time and money, which I prefer.
3. *Human resources:* Hiring and training is a costly and time-intensive processes. If you're one of the lucky ones that every hire stays with you for 40 years, then congratulations! For most of us, life can be unpredictable and employee and practice needs change, leading to dreaded employee turnover. Employees can make or break your practice, which is why it is so important. They are the first face patients see when they walk in and the last they see when they leave. Those interactions are so important. The hiring process is simply the beginning; it is the training that makes a good practice great.

In practice, you cannot handle everything on your own. You will be tied up in the operating room or handling something else and need your staff to act on your behalf. It is therefore important that your employees are "extensions of you": sharing your same desire of delivering top-notch care and handling things in the same manner you would. We have a goal that any patient should be able to ask a question and should get the same answer from whomever they ask.

Fred G. Fedok

I see this question as inquiring about not only what challenges there are, but also what opportunities exist. Our overall goal in the practice is to provide high-quality, contemporary facial plastic surgery care in a relaxed, semi-rural, semi-beachy community.

1. *Time management* has always been viewed as one of the most important facets of my professional life. Clinical volume; clinical production; time for community and social engagement; and time for the family, sleep, and recreation are all in the mix. I prioritize. I take advantage of computer-based to-do lists and reminders for long-range planning. I anticipate and stick to the plan, with various blocks of time remaining fairly constant week to week. Overall, this is been working out very well. I remain busy as well as enjoying a fairly stress-free life.
2. *Delegation* of any and all possible business and practice tasks is an essential. One of the many truths of my professional life is that you cannot do it all yourself. Delegation lives along several different spectrums. Trust, ability, training, and appropriateness are among the considerations. For example, you

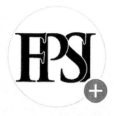

242 **8,013** **2,001**
Posts Followers Following

Jordan Rihani, MD FACS
Plastic Surgeon
Facial Plastic Surgery Institute
Board Certified Facial Plastic Surgeon
🏠 Ft Worth and Southlake TX
☎ (817) 529-3232... more
facialplasticsurgeryinstitute.com
521 W Southlake Blvd, # 175, Southlake, Texas

| Edit Profile | Promotions | Contact |

New   Teaching   Media   Rhinoplasty   Face

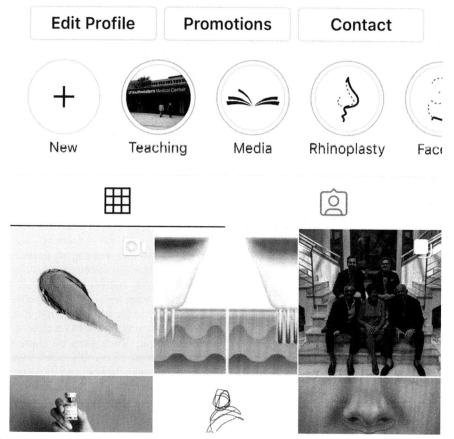

Fig. 6. Rihani Instagram profile.

can only delegate to those who are trained to follow through on the particular task. Obviously as a surgeon, the vast majority of the clinical tasks are performed by me. As the sole clinician in the practice, every other nonclinical aspect or ancillary function may

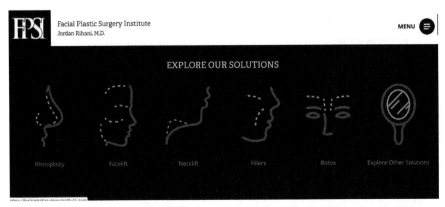

Fig. 7. Rihani Facial Plastic Surgery Institute.

be delegated to trained trusted personnel. Everyone in the office is part of the team. Everyone in the office is well aware of their role and responsibilities in the team. Everybody has a valuable position in the group, and we try to capitalize on their talents or interest to match what is being delegated to them.Frank communication and message reinforcement are necessary. We have frequent meetings where everybody has input to discuss what is working and what's not working. When a process that was developed to handle a specific task is found not to work, we change it.

3. *Attention to the detail of each patient experience.* It all revolves around the patient experience. The patient's personal experience in a medical office is many times in uncharted territory for them. We make every effort to minimize the "unknowns" for patients. We have developed many processes and principles to minimize hassles and wait times for the patient while they are in the office. It is not only what we do, but what the patient perceives as what we do. In our office, our goal is to create a unique optimal patient experience where everybody is regarded as a valuable "family" member. Each patient is treated with the utmost care and respect to get them from point a to point z in their "care" experience. The entire staff is dedicated to making it such. They get it. It is the culture of the office, and the staff have been integral to the creation of our values and culture. We believe we continue to be successful in this endeavor, as we get frequent compliments from patients and outside practices that our office functions better than any other medical setting they have been exposed to.

QUESTION 2. IN YOUR PARTICULAR PRACTICE SETTING, HOW ARE YOU ABLE TO MAINTAIN A LIFE-WORK BALANCE? WHAT DO YOU DEFINE AS YOUR LIFE-WORK BALANCE? HOW DO YOU KEEP FROM WORKING ALL THE TIME? WHAT ARE YOUR STRATEGIES TO PREVENT DISRUPTIONS OF THE BALANCE?
Jessyka G. Lighthall

I define a work-life balance as successfully maintaining a rewarding high-quality clinical practice, performing and publishing research, teaching, continuing my personal education, maintaining personal wellness by staying physically healthy, and spending quality time with family and friends. Admittedly, I have not yet mastered this balance.

Studies evaluating why surgeons leave academic practice to pursue other opportunities found frustration in the academic environment, including a lack of autonomy, administrative burden, challenges fulfilling all facets of an academic practice (research, clinical productivity, teaching), and inability to maintain a healthy work-life balance were recurrent themes.

I have had to narrow the scope of my practice and limit the number of certain cases I do.[2–4]

For example, there were so many rhinoplasty consults that all of my OR block time would be filled months in advance and more urgent cases were being added on to my academic time or were scheduled into the evening hours. By limiting the number of rhinoplasties scheduled per day, I was able to decrease the number of academic days I was operating and leave the hospital at a more acceptable hour to allow quality time with my family. An additional compromise I have had to make is to limit the number of free tissue transfers I perform and now focus on free flaps for facial reanimation.

Although there are some exceptions, for the most part I leave my work at the office and dedicate time away from the hospital to my family. If I do have conference calls or need to check e-mails, they are typically scheduled later in the evening when the family is asleep. I try to limit the number of evening work engagements I attend and am more particular about which courses/conferences I select for continuing medical education.

Finally, to prevent disruptions in this balance, I try to "check-in" with myself at least once per month (it's on my calendar) to review how I am doing, how my family feels things are going, and make necessary adjustments (**Fig. 8**)

Jordan Rihani

For me, the 2 keys to life-work balance are to (1) enjoy work and (2) be possessive of your free time. Enjoying work sounds simple because you love doing surgery, but do you love everything that the workday of a business entails? It can definitely wear on you over time. Anything you can do to create a healthy and positive work environment is not only good for your health but good for the health of your business. Finding energetic, motivated employees that bring different energies and skill sets has allowed me to achieve that balance in the workplace. Second, being possessive of my free time means I try to "leave work at work." I try to do as much as possible while I am there and enjoy my free time off. I did not take calls starting out because I was able to cover my costs without risking additional burnout from late nights in the emergency room (ER). This is an individual decision based on your financial needs and practice goals. Because I didn't have a family to care for,

I was okay making less money for the sake of fewer ER calls. This may not be the correct choice for everyone, but is one that allowed me to focus on other uses of my time. Another simple way I increased my free time was shortening my commute. The time savings of an extra hour a day allowed me to work out regularly and spend more time with friends and family.

Preventing disruptions in the balance for me has been achieved by controlling my work scheduling and avoiding surprises during the day. The 2 scheduling keys for me are (1) grouping appointment types and (2) creating blocks in my schedule. One example of appointment-type grouping is that we try to schedule our regular neurotoxin patients on Monday afternoons. This allows us to rapidly treat 20 plus patients without having to mentally regroup and adjust to be in consult mode or surgical follow-up mode. It creates a flow in the day that feels enjoyable. The second key has been schedule blocks that we usually reserve in the morning or at the end of the day. This allows last-minute flexibility for adding on urgent consults or surgeries without overloading me or my employees. If these blocks don't fill, then it allows us to work on other items to get caught up or call and check on patients.

Fred G. Fedok

For me life-work balance is defined as being engaged with what I want to be engaged in when I want to. This is admittedly because I am the head of the practice and it is a quite different dynamic than when I was in academics with several layers of administration above me. I have the ability to set the tempo of this smaller practice setting.

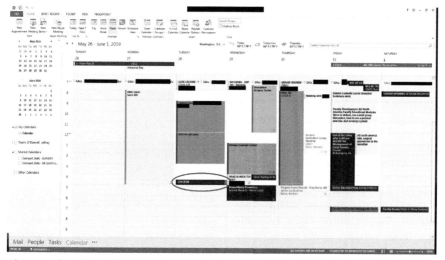

Fig. 8. Rihani screen shot: http://facialplasticsurgeryinstitute.com/-Lighthall calendar.

How this is accomplished really goes back to my answers to question number 1. In this practice, as it is designed, I am fortunate to work the hours I want to work. I work the number of days a week I want to work and practice the particular facets of facial plastic surgery I want to. Although maintained by other people, the daily and weekly schedules are overseen closely by me. In addition, longer-range planning is among the survival habits that I have developed. My wife and I know when we are going on vacation. We know when we are visiting family. We know all of this far in advance. Admittedly, my goals and stresses are different, if not less complex, than they were 30 years ago.

QUESTION 3. HOW DID RESIDENCY AND FELLOWSHIP PREPARE YOU (OR NOT PREPARE YOU) FOR YOUR CURRENT PRACTICE SETTING AND STYLE? WHAT OTHER MENTORING OR TRAINING DO/DID YOU TAKE ADVANTAGE OF?
Jessyka G. Lighthall

My residency and fellowship training prepared me very well for the variety and complexity of cases I see in my practice, as well as juggling multiple academic requirements (eg, research, teaching). Although coming out of training I felt prepared to teach learners of all levels, this has proved more challenging and I have spent time with institutional and national faculty development programs learning about different learning styles, identifying my weaknesses as a teacher, and attempting to optimize my skills as a teacher.

Fellowship did provide some exposure to the "business side" of medicine; however, I felt poorly prepared from a business-management focus, as I did not anticipate I would find myself in management roles having to navigate the nuances of personalities, politics, limited resources, staff turnover, practice finances, and reconciling personal goals with that of the institution/department. I have had to seek out additional faculty development opportunities to learn how to navigate these issues and continue to learn on a daily basis how to be a physician, scribe, coder, professor/educator, manager, marketer, and clinical researcher.

I have sought out mentors locally and nationally, reached out to my fellowship director, and have participated in the American Academy of Facial Plastic and Reconstructive Surgery Mentor for Success Program. These mentors have a wealth of knowledge and wisdom and have been extremely valued in guiding me through my personal and professional development.

Jordan Rihani

My practice environment is modeled on many of the things I witnessed in my facial plastic surgery fellowship. My fellowship directors had a keen understanding of what their cosmetic patients wanted and needed before and after surgery. The attention to detail around the office and their interactions with patients were by far the most important lessons learned throughout my training to prepare me for where I am today.

Residency provided the foundation of the skills that allow me to perform at a high level. My time in training developed skills, such as fundamental surgical techniques, navigation of stressful or overwhelming situations, efficient management of high-volume clinic days, and providing the knowledge base of facial plastic surgery. I continue to refine and build on that skill set every day.

Fred G. Fedok

My residency and training and subsequent clinical experience during my days in academics and previous private practice are all part of the accumulated experiences that I had before opening the private practice. All have been helpful. The clinical experiences, especially with many of the challenges presented within an academic practice, have prepared me for every day in my private practice. A noteworthy aspect of the private practice is that one has to consider not only one's personal clinical acumen when presented with an "interesting" complicated case, but also your available infrastructure and available resources. The "case" that you may have rightfully done in the academic setting may best be referred to a larger center for management. One must try to be cognizant of limitations.

On the administrative side, personnel management, professional issues, financial, and all other nonclinical facets of private practice have been fortunately "learned" by me in my past business and my organizational duties in academic medicine. In private practice there are some differences, but the principles are the same.

QUESTION 4. IN YOUR PARTICULAR PRACTICE, WHAT ARE YOUR HUMAN RESOURCE CHALLENGES, THAT IS, STAFF RETENTION, RECRUITING, TRAINING, HIRING, FIRING. HOW DO YOU MANAGE THEM?
Jessyka G. Lighthall

Staff recruitment and retention is a key human resource challenge in my practice. Several survey studies of academic plastic and facial plastic surgeons have reported that a sense of lack of control of their practices, insufficient staff, and staff retention issues as reasons for decreased job satisfaction.[2–4] For most of my academic practice, physicians have had minimal input into who is hired, reporting of performance measures, compensation changes, scope of practice, or termination of employees. In addition, the recruitment and hiring process is often so drawn out that there is a constant cycle of understaffed positions, overworking of existing staff, and therefore lack of retention of employees with frequent turnover. This creates a sense of lack of control of my practice environment and a feeling of constant flux. With multiple issues with turnover that have directly impacted my practice and patients, I have been able to be more involved and interview staff that will hold key positions for my practice (eg, surgery scheduler). However, most of these human resources challenges still exist.

Jordan Rihani

My biggest human resources challenge starting a new practice has been finding the right employees and training them to be extensions of yourself. It is one of the most important decisions you can make and one of my biggest time investments. The best way to manage people is to be humble, professional, consistent, and maintain open communication. If you set the tone early that everyone should speak their mind and keep them from feeling scared to speak their mind, the workplace will be more egalitarian and you may receive feedback you wouldn't otherwise receive until that employee has decided to pack their bags.

You should understand your staff and their personalities so that you can place them in the correct roles to optimize their strengths. An obvious example is that someone with a bubbly, talkative personality is great for a front-facing position. The employee who works hard but doesn't smile is probably not the person who should be greeting patients on their arrival.

There are a few tips I have found create a more relaxed work environment. The first is to hire one more employee than I actually need. This allows me to adjust when an employee may be out on vacation or sick. Not to mention, there is always something to do in a growing practice. Second, I enjoy building team rapport with regular after-work social outings, which can make for a more relaxed work environment. Once this work environment has been created, overall stress level decreases substantially. There are tense times, as there would be in any workplace or family, it is how you communicate and work through

problems that ultimately determines how successful you will be.

Fred G. Fedok

The general principles regarding human resource issues are largely the same in all professional settings. The general principles were the same in my academic practice as in my current private practice. The general laws governing labor relations are fairly consistent from state to state. The current accepted norms of workplace behavior are the same from industry to industry. The major difference in my experience is the locus and proximity of control and the policies and procedures for the management of human resource matters. The biggest variable is the culture of the practice. In private practice you have the incredible ability to create. Hire good people. Hire people with the right fit and comparable values. Honesty and a willingness to learn are essentials. Their fit and values are in many ways more important than the "numbers" they generate. If a particular employee's work productivity is lacking, make a change in their duties and responsibilities to see if they can be adapted into the practice. Take the time to communicate with them before it becomes an emotionally charged issue. If an acceptable change is not possible, unfortunately one may have to terminate the relationship. I have always felt one can consider your staff with the idea that each member is a collection of positive and negative work-related attributes. In your organization, if your value the employee, your challenge as supervisor is to find where their particular talent may be the most help in the organization. If there is not a match, then unfortunately, they may have to be let go. It will be better for all involved.

QUESTION 5. WHAT ARE SOME OF THE ADVANTAGES YOU PERCEIVE TO "YOUR OPPOSITE STYLE OF PRACTICE": WHAT ARE SOME OF THE CHALLENGES THAT YOU EXPERIENCE IN YOUR PRACTICE ENVIRONMENT THAT YOU THINK ARE LESS FRUSTRATING IN A DIFFERENT ENVIRONMENT?
Jessyka G. Lighthall

A recently published survey of academic facial plastic surgeons and department chairs reported desire for more control of practice as being the primary reason that academic facial plastic surgeons reported leaving their current practice, and providing more control as a key[3] maneuver to improve faculty retention. This study also found reasons that surgeons left academic practice were to improve their compensation, obtain the ability to market their practice, and have an off-site location for aesthetic patients, which private practice affords.

Although I have never practiced outside the academic environment, I expect that private practice allows for a higher degree of autonomy and control of the practice environment. Specifically, more control over staff/nursing recruitment and retention to identify personnel that are a good fit for the practice and it nuances, providing additional training, and setting competitive market compensation to recruit top applicants.

Although not universally true, there is in general a higher earning potential for physicians outside of the academic setting but also an increased financial risk without a salary guarantee of the academic environment. Control over marketing is improved within a private practice, as is the utilization of social media.

Without the academic requirements of teaching medical students and residents or performing research unless there is a specific interest, this likely allows more energy to be focused on building a productive and efficient clinical practice and maintaining work-life balance.

Jordan Rihani

In my opinion, a practice in academics is beneficial for 3 types of people: those interested in research and publishing, those trying to build a national or international reputation, and those whose primary passion is teaching. Although I love teaching and do it regularly in my practice, it is not something I do daily. At this time in my life, my primary passion is performing surgery and delivering high-quality outcomes. Allowing residents to perform the surgeries and educate on that level would be difficult with my current primary objectives. From a research standpoint, having access to institutional resources and residents facilitates easier production of clinical and basic science research and publications. This allows for higher volume publications, which can boost your reputation as an academician. I have found my own balance with teaching, working with injectable companies as well as affiliating with a local academic program to work with residents. Those relationships have also allowed residents to come out to my practice to watch and learn when desired.

I think any practice environment has its pros and cons, many of which center around control. If you like controlling every detail, then you may not want to be in an environment in which you need institutional approval to make changes. It is really just understanding what you want your practice to look like and pick what practice setting you need

to do to get to that point. Don't make it a financial decision, for example, you need a little more money now and want a salary or that you need a little more security with benefits. Those are probably the wrong reasons to make the academic versus private practice decision.

Fred G. Fedok

This question allows me to highlight some of the differences between academic and private practice along several parameters I believe are important.

Mentoring and collegiality

I am a firm believer that most persons finishing medical training are best served by entering academic practice or a healthy private practice where there can be some early oversight and mentoring provided to aid the individual in decision making and some technical assistance. I believe that some of the most unfortunate complications that were sent into us at the university were situations that may have been avoided had the young surgeon been in a situation in which mentoring and guidance had been available to them. Usually the larger number of faculty in an academic practice allows more opportunity for oversight and mentoring. This is an especially important issue for the developing clinician.

Research

I am currently the lead investigator for a Food and Drug Administration investigation of a medical device. Those opportunities are rather limited in private practice for a variety of reasons. If one truly has a talent and a desire to do credible research, it is fundamentally easier in an academic or in a larger corporate setting.

Scholarly engagement, organizational engagement, program development

A core aspect of academic surgical practice is the encouragement and incentivizing the engagement of the individual to develop leadership positions in scholarly and organizational pursuits.

Autonomy/responsibility

Private practice offers more opportunities for independent decision making and for shaping the trajectory and focus of the practice. In a larger practice, especially an academic practice, the goals are established on a larger collective basis. There is an inverse relationship between Autonomy and Responsibility; the more autonomy one exercises, the more risk and responsibility one is also assuming. Both practice settings have advantages and disadvantages for the individual.

How long to stay in academic practice? How about "long enough" as an answer. For each individual there is an answer.

QUESTION 6. WHAT IS MOST ENJOYABLE ABOUT YOUR PRACTICE? WHAT IS THE LEAST ENJOYABLE? WHAT ARE THE TOP BENEFITS AND TOP DRAWBACKS TO YOUR PRACTICE TYPE? WHAT KEEPS YOU IN YOUR CURRENT PRACTICE STYLE?
Jessyka G. Lighthall

Although many of these have been mentioned previously, the least enjoyable aspects of academic practice are the excessive administrative duties, dealing with the electronic medical record, lack of control of my practice environment, slow pace at which change or improvements occur, and difficulties maintaining my work-life balance.

The most enjoyable aspects of my career are the patients, the high complexity and variety of cases, and ability to educate medical students and train residents. I also enjoy the collegiality and camaraderie within the department and institution as a whole. Other benefits of academic practice are having a consistent salary, opportunity for career advancement, and the availability of funds for continual medical education or faculty development. Health benefits are provided, malpractice and disability insurance are covered, and a retirement savings program is also available.

There is no perfect practice setting and surgeons may move through these environments as they mature in their practices and reprioritize competing interests.

Jordan Rihani

The most enjoyable part of my practice is being in the operating room and doing what I love: surgery. That is why I went into this field in the first place and that stands true today. I genuinely enjoy making people feel better about themselves and improving their quality of life. I have a great staff and, as a result, great patients.

The least enjoyable part of my practice is probably the social media and content creation! I find it to be rather time-consuming and, although important, not something I am particularly interested in. Top benefit/drawback of my practice setup as a private solo practitioner is that it is a high-risk, high-reward scenario. If you do not make money, then you don't get to write yourself a check. Everyone gets paid first: your employees, creditors, landlords, and suppliers. The trade-off is that there is a direct financial compensation based on your performance. Everything you earn above your expenses is yours to keep. For this reason,

combined with time flexibility, I really enjoy my practice style. I am not accountable to anyone else for my financial or practice decisions. In other words, I love being my own boss. I control everything, which can be stressful, but also a huge advantage when trying to build your practice.

Fred G. Fedok

I intensely enjoy several aspects about my current practice situation. The ability to provide a beneficial service to patients is at the core of the satisfaction. This includes both cosmetic and functional realms of care. There are many components of the practice and local social environment that make this possible. As mentioned earlier, it is really a group effort within the practice that drives this. Everyone in the office is on-board in propelling our practice engagement philosophy forward. That is really one of the enjoyable features: to make it work and see it take form. To get the positive feedback from patients is to compel one even to do it better. The design and evolution of the practice is for me the new interesting project that is being developed and honed. As I was able to do so in academics, I am able to do it again in a different location and manner.

There are few perceived drawbacks. Conceptually being part of a larger private or academic practice would suggest the availability of more resources. Inherently, though, there would be less autonomy and that would interfere in our proposed practice trajectory.

SUMMARY

We believe it is most appropriate that we allow the reader to draw their own conclusions about what has been written here. Some general principles of the differences in academic versus private practice have been highlighted. The individual experiences of the authors have lent real-life insight into these differences and similarities. As one does future planning about their own career, we encourage you to research these dynamics in the same way that one invests time and research in planning the management of any complex surgical issue. We are confident that most facial plastic surgeons will be open to sharing perspective on their life as a facial plastic surgeon.

DISCLOSURE

The authors have nothing to disclose.

REFERENCES

1. Khansa I, Janis JE. A growing epidemic: plastic surgeons and burnout - a literature review. Plast Reconstr Surg 2019;144(2):298e–305e.
2. Jumaily JS, Spiegel JH. The unique practice needs of academic facial plastic and reconstructive surgeons. JAMA Facial Plast Surg 2015;17(5):384–5.
3. Kowalczyk DM, Jordan JR. Facial plastic surgery faculty turnover: survey of academic facial plastic surgeons and department chairs. Int Arch Otorhinolaryngol 2019;23(2):209–17.
4. Chen JT, Girotto JA, Kitzmiller WJ, et al. Academic plastic surgery: faculty recruitment and retention. Plast Reconstr Surg 2014;133(3):393e–404e.

How to Leverage Social Media in Private Practice

Thuy-Van T. Ho, MD[a],*, Steven H. Dayan, MD[b]

KEYWORDS

- Social media • Private practice • Facial plastic surgery • Instagram • Facebook • YouTube
- Snapchat • Twitter

KEY POINTS

- Social media platforms are useful for marketing, professional networking, patient and surgeon education, and personal and professional support.
- Prospective patients increasingly are turning to social media applications to perform their research on cosmetic treatments and plastic surgeons.
- Social media engagement is particularly high among young adults, who are now more commonly seeking cosmetic treatments for early care and prejuvenation.
- Facial plastic surgeons who engage in social media need to adequately understand both the benefits and challenges to social media for translated success to their practice.

INTRODUCTION

Since the advent of the Internet, health care information has become increasingly more accessible. According to the Pew Research Center, approximately half of Americans were using the Internet in 2000, and that number has jumped to 9 in 10 Americans as of 2019.[1]

Furthermore, the number of Americans who rely on smartphones as their primary venue of home online access is increasing. Today, 1 in 5 Americans are smartphone-only Internet users, with reliance on smartphones for online access particularly common among younger adults, nonwhites, and lower-income Americans.[1] Social media, which can be defined as any interactive Internet-based applications that facilitate the creation and sharing of information, ideas, messages, and other means of expression, often for purposes of social networking, now dominates the current online landscape. Since 2018, a majority of American adults use Facebook (69%) and YouTube (73%).[2,3] Among younger adults ages 18 years to 24 years old, 78% utilize Snapchat, whereas 71% use Instagram.[2]

Facial plastic surgeons in private practice need to recognize the rising influence of social media as it extends to the realm of facial plastic surgery. Social media platforms are useful for professional networking, patient and surgeon education, and personal and professional support.[4] Moreover, patients in the modern era commonly utilize the Internet and relevant Web site applications to perform research on conditions and treatments of interest as well as on potential surgeons before they walk in the door for a consultation. Although aesthetic medicine is widely accepted as a consumer-driven field, it also is important to recognize that health care in general is trending in a similar direction. Facial plastic surgeons in this current era who demonstrate a good understanding of the potentials as well as pitfalls of social media can then harness this online avenue to their advantage and ultimately be more successful in their practice. This article reviews the most recent trends in social media and facial plastic surgery and the benefits and challenges of social media in private practice as well as concrete tips for the private practice facial plastic surgeon for

[a] Rejuvenation Medical Aesthetics, 451 South State Street, Suite C, Newtown, PA 18940, USA; [b] Division of Facial Plastic and Reconstructive Surgery, Department of Otolaryngology, Chicago Center for Facial Plastic Surgery, University of Illinois at Chicago, 845 North Michigan Avenue, Suite 923E, Chicago, IL 60611, USA
* Corresponding author.
E-mail address: thuyvantinaho@gmail.com

Facial Plast Surg Clin N Am 28 (2020) 515–522
https://doi.org/10.1016/j.fsc.2020.07.002
1064-7406/20/© 2020 Elsevier Inc. All rights reserved.

taking advantage of the most popular social media platforms (Instagram, YouTube, Facebook, Snapchat, and Twitter).

TRENDS IN SOCIAL MEDIA

According to the Pew Research Center, the social media landscape in 2018 was "defined by a mix of long-standing trends and newly emerging narratives" and has remained mostly unchanged in 2019.[2,3] The steady growth of adoption of social media in the United States over the past decade actually has been slowing down, with the numbers of American adults who use Facebook, Pinterest, LinkedIn, and Twitter remaining largely the same since 2016.[3] As stated previously, a majority of adults in the United States subscribe to Facebook and YouTube (**Fig. 1**). On the other hand, there has been an increase in the number of Instagram users, particularly with younger adults. Among younger adults ages 18 years to 24 years old, Snapchat and Instagram are extremely popular and used by the majority, which reflects a substantial age-related difference in social media platform preferences (**Fig. 2**). Furthermore, there exists an overarching notable difference in social media use by age. Although 88% of 18 year olds to 29 year olds endorse engaging in any form of social media, this number falls to 78% of 30 year olds to 49 year olds, to 64% of 50 year olds to 64 year olds, and to 37% of adults 65 years old and older.[2]

Among Americans who subscribe to social media applications, a majority of these users engage in these applications daily. As of 2019%, 74% of Facebook users visit the Web site daily, with half of these users doing so several times per day (**Fig. 3**). A majority of Snapchat and Instagram users visit these applications daily as well, especially in the 18-year-old to 24-year-old age group. According to the Pew Research Center, among younger adult Americans, 77% of Snapchat subscribers use the application daily, including 68% who engage with the application multiple times per day. The corresponding numbers for Instagram users ages 18 years to 24 years old are 76% and 60%, respectively.[3]

In their 2018 study, the Pew Research Center also found a trend of substantial reciprocity across major social media platforms (**Fig. 4**). Of the assessed social media platforms (Twitter, Instagram, Facebook, Snapchat, YouTube, WhatsApp, Pinterest, and LinkedIn), 73% engage in more than 1 social media application, and the median American uses 3 of these 8 platforms.[2] The median 18 year old to 29 year old utilizes 4 of these platforms. **Fig. 5** illustrates an additional breakdown of

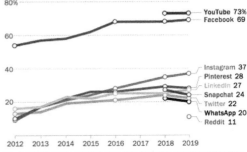

Facebook, YouTube continue to be the most widely used online platforms among U.S. adults

% of U.S. adults who say they ever use the following online platforms or messaging apps online or on their cellphone

Note: Pre-2018 telephone poll data is not available for YouTube, Snapchat and WhatsApp. Comparable trend data is not available for Reddit.
Source: Survey conducted Jan. 8-Feb. 7, 2019.

PEW RESEARCH CENTER

Fig. 1. A majority of adults use Facebook and Twitter. (*From* Share of U.S adults using social media, including Facebook, is mostly unchanged since 2018. Pewinternet.org. https://www.pewresearch.org/fact-tank/2019/04/10/share-of-u-s-adults-using-social-media-including-facebook-is-mostly-unchanged-since-2018/. Published April 10, 2019. Accessed August 17, 2019; with permission.)

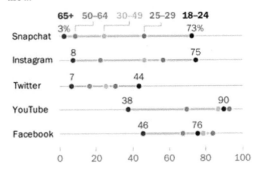

Snapchat and Instagram are especially popular among 18- to 24-y-olds

% of U.S. adults in each age group who say they ever use ...

Note: Respondents who did not give an answer are not shown.
Source: Survey conducted Jan. 8-Feb. 7, 2019.

PEW RESEARCH CENTER

Fig. 2. Snapchat and Instagram popularity among 18 year olds to 24 year olds. (*From* Share of U.S adults using social media, including Facebook, is mostly unchanged since 2018. Pewinternet.org. https://www.pewresearch.org/fact-tank/2019/04/10/share-of-u-s-adults-using-social-media-including-facebook-is-mostly-unchanged-since-2018/. Published April 10, 2019. Accessed August 17, 2019; with permission.)

Roughly three-quarters of Facebook users visit the site on a daily basis

Among U.S. adults who say they use ___, % who use each site ...

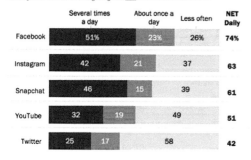

Note: Respondents who did not give an answer are not shown. "Less often" category includes users who visit these sites a few times a week, every few weeks or less often.
Source: Survey conducted Jan. 8-Feb. 7, 2019.

PEW RESEARCH CENTER

Fig. 3. A majority of Facebook users utilize the site daily. (*From* Share of U.S adults using social media, including Facebook, is mostly unchanged since 2018. Pewinternet.org. https://www.pewresearch.org/fact-tank/2019/04/10/share-of-u-s-adults-using-social-media-including-facebook-is-mostly-unchanged-since-2018/. Published April 10, 2019. Accessed August 17, 2019; with permission.)

different social media platform use by various demographic groups as well.

Plastic surgeons have come to appreciate the building impact of social media and increasingly are adapting social media platforms into their practice. A 2019 online survey of American Society of Plastic Surgeons members revealed that 61.9% endorsed having an active professional social media account.[5] Among those surgeons with a practice primarily devoted to aesthetic surgery, 79.4% responded they had an active professional social media account. Overall, the study concluded that younger surgeons in private practice were more likely to view social media as an acceptable avenue of reaching patients,[5] which parallels the trends in social media use by age.

TRENDS IN FACIAL PLASTIC SURGERY PATIENTS

Prospective patients seeking aesthetic treatments currently rely heavily on the Internet and increasingly more so on social media applications to research and find their plastic surgeons. A 2019 study by the Department of Plastic and Reconstructive Surgery at Georgetown University and the Division of Plastic and Reconstructive Surgery at Mount Sinai Health System assessing public preferences on plastic surgery social media engagement and professionalism found Google to be the first source where individuals look for a plastic surgeon (46%).[6] When survey respondents were asked regarding the most influential online methods for choosing a surgeon, social media platforms as a whole

Substantial 'reciprocity' across major social media platforms

% of ___ users who also ...

	Use Twitter	Use Instagram	Use Facebook	Use Snapchat	Use YouTube	Use WhatsApp	Use Pinterest	Use LinkedIn
Twitter	--	73%	90%	54%	95%	35%	49%	50%
Instagram	50	--	91	60	95	35	47	41
Facebook	32	47	--	35	87	27	37	33
Snapchat	48	77	89	--	95	33	44	37
YouTube	31	45	81	35	--	28	36	32
WhatsApp	38	55	85	40	92	--	33	40
Pinterest	41	56	89	41	92	25	--	42
LinkedIn	47	57	90	40	94	35	49	--

Source: Survey conducted Jan. 3-10, 2018.
"Social Media Use in 2018"

90% of LinkedIn users also use Facebook

PEW RESEARCH CENTER

Fig. 4. Substantial reciprocity across social media platforms. (*From* Social media use in 2018. Pewinternet.org. https://www.pewinternet.org/2018/03/01/social-media-use-in-2018/. Published March 1, 2018. Accessed August 17, 2019; with permission.)

Use of different online platforms by demographic groups

% of US adults who say they ever use the following online platforms or messaging apps

	YouTube	Facebook	Instagram	Pinterest	LinkedIn	Snapchat	Twitter	WhatsApp	Reddit
US adults	73%	69%	37%	28%	27%	24%	22%	20%	11%
Men	78	63	31	15	29	24	24	21	15
Women	68	75	43	42	24	24	21	19	8
White	71	70	33	33	28	22	21	13	12
Black	77	70	40	27	24	28	24	24	4
Hispanic	78	69	51	22	16	29	25	42	14
Ages 18-29	91	79	67	34	28	62	38	23	22
18–24	90	76	75	38	17	73	44	20	21
25–29	93	84	57	28	44	47	31	28	23
30–49	87	79	47	35	37	25	26	31	14
50–64	70	68	23	27	24	9	17	16	6
65+	38	46	8	15	11	3	7	3	1
<$30,000	68	69	35	18	10	27	20	19	9
$30,000-$74,999	75	72	39	27	26	26	20	16	10
$75,000+	83	74	42	41	49	22	31	25	15
High school or less	64	61	33	19	9	22	13	18	6
Some college	79	75	37	32	26	29	24	14	14
College+	80	74	43	38	51	20	32	28	15
Urban	77	73	46	30	33	29	26	24	11
Suburban	74	69	35	30	30	20	22	19	13
Rural	64	66	21	26	10	20	13	10	8

Note: Respondents who did not give an answer are not shown. Whites and blacks include only non-Hispanics. Hispanics are of any race.
Source: Survey conducted Jan. 8-Feb. 7, 2019.

PEW RESEARCH CENTER

Fig. 5. Social media use by different demographic groups. (*From* Share of U.S adults using social media, including Facebook, is mostly unchanged since 2018. Pewinternet.org. https://www.pewresearch.org/fact-tank/2019/04/10/share-of-u-s-adults-using-social-media-including-facebook-is-mostly-unchanged-since-2018/. Published April 10, 2019. Accessed August 17, 2019; with permission.)

ranked highest (35%) followed by practice Web site (25%). Those participants who were considering surgical or nonsurgical procedures were 3 times more likely to pick social media platforms as the most influential online method behind surgeon choice and 5 times more likely to follow a plastic surgeon on social media. Moreover, 96% of respondents were unclear regarding the type of board certification that should be held by a plastic surgeon.[6] It also has been shown that total number of social media followers, and not medical school ranking and years in practice,

was associated significantly with Google front-page placement.[7]

The American Academy of Facial Plastic and Reconstructive Surgery 2018 annual survey also discovered that the cosmetic patient population is extending younger. The survey findings showed a "strong link between Millennials (now 22–37 years old) and the growing demand for cosmetic procedures," with more emphasis on early care and prejuvenation in the 20s and 30s age range.[8] Surgical procedures on average are up 47% and botulinum toxin injections have increased by 22% since 2013. In 2018%, 72% of facial plastic surgeons noted an increase in cosmetic surgery or injectables in patients under age 30, which is a significant increase from 2017 and up 24% from 2013.[8] It is important for facial plastic surgeons to embrace the rising millennial patient population and their major involvement in social media, because this age group finds plastic surgery more normalized and mainstream via social media content and, therefore, invests in facial rejuvenation sooner.

BENEFITS OF SOCIAL MEDIA IN PRIVATE PRACTICE
Social Media Augments Marketing Potential

The use of social media has several advantages for facial plastic surgeons in private practice. First, social media platforms provide an additional avenue for facial plastic surgeons to market themselves and their services. Although engagement in certain social media applications, such as Instagram and YouTube, can be time consuming, the commitment often comes with much less financial cost especially compared with Web site maintenance and more traditional channels of marketing, such as print. Facial plastic surgeons more readily can showcase treatment specials, before-and-after photographs, patient reviews, and even live demonstrations of procedures to appeal more to prospective patients.

Social Media Offers a Window to the Personal Side of the Surgeon

In addition, the close interactivity of social media platforms offers facial plastic surgeons the opportunity to demonstrate more their personality, which in turn may help attract potential patients beyond their credentials and photographed results. A 2019 study based on an Instagram social experiment featuring a created account called "doctor.aesthetics" revealed that scientific posts yielded low response rate, whereas private posts were associated with a significantly enhanced number of likes and led to the most clicks and new followers.[9]

Social Media Provides an Education Platform

Furthermore, social media can offer an education platform for facial plastic surgeons. Depending on the priorities of individual surgeons, they may consider putting out informative content posts, videos, blogs, and question-and-answer forums to educate as well as engage consumer followers regarding particular facial conditions or concerns as well as treatments, especially in the realm of aesthetic medicine. These types of educational efforts can help reduce stigmas and reverse incorrect perceptions about nonsurgical and surgical rejuvenation procedures as well as reinforce to prospective patients the importance of safe protocols by adequately trained professionals. Facial plastic surgeons who establish themselves as knowledgeable experts on social media platforms in turn enhance their marketability to potential patients as well.

Social Media Promotes Opportunities for Self-Learning and Networking

Social media also be can utilized by facial plastic surgeons as means of furthering their own education as well as social networking. The opportunity to follow and engage other professionals in an intimate real-time online platform facilitates immediate exchange of ideas and knowledge. A facial plastic surgeon who engages in social media can use this avenue to learn more about procedural tips and techniques from other surgeons, the latest trends in innovative technology, and marketing campaigns by other practices. Facial plastic surgeons also can interact and communicate more quickly via social media and subsequently build relationships, with increased opportunities for networking and mentorship. According to a 2018 study centered on a survey investigating trainee and physician social media use, respondents in surgical subspecialties were more likely to report engaging in social media to build a network of same-sex mentorship.[10] This finding is particularly applicable to female surgeons, who may have less opportunity for same-sex mentors at their own institutions.

CHALLENGES OF SOCIAL MEDIA IN PRIVATE PRACTICE
Information Through Social Media Is Unregulated and Not Always Accurate

Although health information is much more accessible and abundant via social media channels, it remains unregulated, with accuracy not guaranteed. Although modern-era patients may be more informed and well-researched, it is the duty of the facial plastic surgeon to gauge patients' level of knowledge and help educate them correctly in consultation regardless of what they learned through social media. As aesthetic medicine continues to gain prominence, the number of health professionals who assert themselves as cosmetic providers also is rising. Prospective patients tapped into social media may more likely subscribe to the platform of a non–board-certified health provider with several thousand followers over facial plastic surgeons and plastic surgeons who formally trained in and are board certified in plastic surgery.

The Number of Unverified or Non–Board-Certified Authorities with Social Media Platforms on Aesthetic Medicine Is Rising

A 2019 study from the Johns Hopkins University Department of Plastic and Reconstructive Surgery on plastic surgery hashtag utilization in social media discovered that among a sample Instagram query of 15 plastic surgery-related hashtags, 75% of posts were by medical professionals with 56% of posts authored by board-certified physicians. Furthermore, nonphysicians (nurse practitioners, physician assistants, or registered nurses) were more likely to post about nonsurgical procedures and injectables, and physicians without training in plastic surgery or otolaryngology were more likely to post nonsurgical procedure–related hashtags.[11] A 2018 study from the Division of Plastic and Reconstructive Surgery at Northwestern found that American Society for Aesthetic Plastic Surgery (ASAPS) eligible board-certified plastic surgeons are underrepresented among physicians submitting top plastic surgery–related content on Instagram. More specifically, the investigators noted from their focused Instagram query that plastic surgeons eligible for ASAPS membership were responsible for only 17.8% of the top posts.[12] In addition, all non–plastic surgery–trained physicians identified from this study marketed themselves as "cosmetic surgeons."

Social Media Possesses Negative Backlash Implications

Although social media applications allow users to engage and interconnect readily in positive ways, this kind of communication remains impersonal and superficial compared with real human-to-human interaction and promotes channels of negative feedback and backlash just as readily. According to a 2018 analysis of key phrases "plastic surgery" and "#plastic_surgery" feature on Instagram, YouTube, and Facebook, the 10 most powerful attention-drawing motives behind social media posts were jokes, attractive female plastic surgeons, celebrities, personal stories, provocative surgeries, videos or photos of surgeries, sex, shaming, and patient education.[13] Celebrity-endorsed posts received the most attention in terms of likes, comments, shares, and views. Facial plastic surgeons also always need to utilize social media with precaution and care, because any social media post leaves lasting imprint in the Internet realm, and patient privacy and professionalism always should be upheld.

INSTAGRAM

Instagram is among the newer social media platforms but is on the rise and is popular particularly among the 18-year-old to 24-year-old age group. It began simply as a medium for sharing picturesque photographs among users but has evolved into so much more. In the current era, Instagram has been used as a channel for individuals to promote a brand based on increased exposure through quantitative numbers of followers and likes. Celebrities are very tuned in to Instagram as are social media influencers who base their careers on building a popular platform following and then getting paid for advertising products and experiences and various kinds of collaborations.

For facial plastic surgeons, Instagram offers a visually appealing and interactive space for marketing their brand and education to prospective patients. Posts that feature before-and-after photos, patient reviews, procedure tips or videos, and even personal content that can be liked or commented on help promote facial plastic surgeons as experts in the craft as well as their personal side to help attract patients. On the surface, a surgeon also may seem more like an authority in their field with a strong following, although this observation should be taken with a grain of salt, because the image an individual or business portrays on Instagram can be deceiving. The story function is a more real-time, interactive feature to Instagram that allows surgeons to show more of themselves and their practice on a day-to-day basis and in turn engage followers more. The Instagram Live (IGTV) feature allows surgeons to post videos of longer duration than a story or post videos that typically are limited to 60 seconds or less. Users who watch posts on IGTV can scroll through and watch videos of other accounts they do not follow. Moreover, Instagram offers excellent opportunities for a surgeon to learn from others and engage in mentorship and networking relationships by following and communicating with other surgeons and aesthetic medicine providers.

FACEBOOK

Facebook is social media Web site centered on individual or group profiles. From a professional standpoint, a facial plastic surgeon may create a business profile page on Facebook that features information regarding the surgeon and the surgeon's offered services and contact information as well as patient photos, educational videos, and even promotions. Facebook offers another opportunity beyond the practice Web site for surgeons to advertise their practice and brand to prospective patients as well as interact with them more quickly. Followers may like or comment on posts and updates and even can book appointments through the Facebook practice page. There also is a Facebook stories section where the surgeon or practice can post more in the moment that lasts only 24 hours on the stories feed. As discussed previously, Facebook remains one of the most popular social media applications across all age groups as a whole and thus can be advantageous in appealing to the broader potential patient population.

Furthermore, if surgeons already have a personal profile page on Facebook, they may consider linking the personal and professional pages, especially in terms of recruiting followers and participation from their established friends network. Facebook as a social media platform also is ideal for social networking, with the ability to find and friend personal friends or colleagues through other friends or even create and/or participate in groups or forums with common interests and goals.

YouTube

YouTube is a social media platform for sharing videos. For the facial plastic surgeon, this medium is a great opportunity to showcase live demonstrations, surgical techniques, patient testimonials, and surgeon personal interviews to promote branding and education for the prospective patient. In contrast to Instagram, where video clips are limited by duration, YouTube can be utilized as a source for posting videos of higher production level. At the same time, however, more time, preparation, and resources may need to be devoted to each post compared with some of the other social media applications. YouTube additionally is a great resource for facial plastic surgeons to learn from other surgeons who previously have posted their own videos on procedural technique and tips.

SNAPCHAT

Snapchat is a social media application that enables users to send their contacts immediate photos or videos captured from their daily life and even post them to their story for all followers to view that are available for viewing for no longer than 24 hours. Like Instagram, Snapchat has become increasingly popular among younger adults ages 18 years to 24 years old. Given that

Instagram also installed a story feature that further boosted user engagement, however, it will be interesting to trend the popularity of Snapchat in the near future. The story feature of Snapchat allows facial plastic surgeons to show more of their personal side in everyday life and ultimately increase their appeal to prospective patients. Facial plastic surgeons in private practice should consider syncing their Snapchat and Instagram accounts such that the story posts are featured on both applications simultaneously or they may prefer to devote more of their time and energy to Instagram based on the degree of overlap between the 2 social media platforms.

TWITTER

Twitter is a social media platform that allows users to rapidly communicate messages in text format, with a limit of total of 140 characters at a time. Images and videos also can be linked with the text posts for heightened impact. From the private practice facial plastic surgeon standpoint, Twitter may be an advantageous medium for those surgeons who are interested in promoting an education platform and in engaging with other colleagues on topics in plastic surgery and aesthetic medicine. Interestingly enough, a 2018 study focused on identifying and assessing the top influencers in plastic surgery on Twitter found that 77% of the top influencers are trained as plastic surgeons or facial plastic surgeons.[14] On the other hand, it is difficult to ascertain how beneficial Twitter engagement may be in patient recruitment, because prospective cosmetic patients typically prefer to view visual photos or videos as part of their research.

SOCIAL MEDIA POSTING TIPS FOR SUCCESS

1. Educate or inspire with every post. Have a purpose behind each post.
2. Post regularly according to follower viewing activity. For Instagram, for example, consider posting to the news feed 2 times to 3 times per week to start and to the story daily.
3. Community engagement is key to growth. Engage on a regular basis with other users (like and comment on other posts; follow other accounts are appealing). Reply to all comments on posts as soon as possible and with meaningful responses for added exposure.
4. Consider hiring professional help, having a staff member help, or using organizational applications to help with 2 and 3, based on time commitments.

5. Consider paying to boost posts on certain social media applications (eg, Instagram and Facebook). Boosted posts are promoted as ads on user feeds that do not already follow an application.
6. Post often, when possible, in video format if not camera-shy. Ensure video content is captivating to attract viewers to a page.
7. Do not be afraid to make personal posts. Often these posts attract the most likes and comments.
8. If engaging in multiple social media platforms, synchronize them so they post the same content simultaneously.
9. Be kind and avoid negativity.

SUMMARY

Social media is a widely popular as well as powerful tool for means of online engagement and interaction. Facial plastic surgeons in private practice should embrace social media as an opportune medium for marketing, patient recruitment, education, and networking. With a thorough knowledge of both the benefits and challenges of social media as well as the current trends in social media and the plastic surgery population, the well-versed and well-equipped facial plastic surgeon can take on social media in a thoughtful manner that will serve to benefit a practice greatly.

DISCLOSURE

The authors certify that they have no affiliations with or involvement in any organization or entity with any financial interest (such as honoraria; educational grants; participation in speakers' bureaus; membership, employment, consultancies, stock ownership, or other equity interest; and expert testimony or patent-licensing arrangements) or nonfinancial interest (such as personal or professional relationships, affiliations, knowledge, or beliefs) in the subject matter or materials discussed in this article.

REFERENCES

1. Demographics of internet and home broadband usage. 2019. Available at: Pewinternet.org; https://www.pewinternet.org/fact-sheet/internet-broadband/. Accessed August 17, 2019.
2. Social media use in 2018. 2018. Available at: Pewinternet.org; https://www.pewinternet.org/2018/03/01/social-media-use-in-2018/. Accessed August 17, 2019.
3. Share of U.S. adults using social media, including Facebook, is mostly unchanged since 2018. 2019. Available at: Pewinternet.org; https://www.pewresearch.org/fact-tank/2019/04/10/share-of-u-s-adults-using-social-media-including-facebook-is-mostly-unchanged-since-2018/. Accessed August 17, 2019.
4. Joshi KG, Gehle ME. The role of social media in private practice. 2019. Available at: Psychiatrictimes.com; https://www.psychiatrictimes.com/special-reports/role-social-media-private-practice/. Accessed August 17, 2019.
5. Dorfman RG, Mahmood E, Ren A, et al. Google ranking of plastic surgeons values social media presence over academic pedigree and experience. Aesthet Surg J 2019;39(4):447–51.
6. Economides JM, Fan KL, Pittman TA. An analysis of plastic surgeons' social media use and perceptions. Aesthet Surg J 2019;39(7):794–802.
7. Fan KL, Graziano F, Economides JM, et al. The public's preferences on plastic surgery social media engagement and professionalism: Demystifying the impact of demographics. Plast Reconstr Surg 2019;143(2):619–30.
8. AAFPRS 2018 annual survey reveals key trends in facial plastic surgery. 2019. Available at: Aafprs.org; https://www.aafprs.org/media/stats_polls/m_stats.html. Accessed August 19, 2019.
9. Klietz ML, Kaiser HW, Machens HG, et al. Social media marketing: What do prospective patients want to see? Aesthet Surg J 2019;40(5):577–83.
10. Luc JG, Stamp NL, Antonoff MB. Social media in the mentorship and networking of physicians: Important role for women in surgical subspecialties. Am J Surg 2018;215(4):752–60.
11. Siegel N, Jenny H, Chopra K, et al. What does it mean to be a #plasticsurgeon? Analyzing plastic surgery hashtag utilization in social media. Aesthet Surg J 2020;40(4):NP213–8.
12. Dorfman RG, Vaca EE, Mahmood E, et al. Plastic surgery-related hashtag utilization on Instagram: implications for education and marketing. Aesthet Surg J 2018;38(3):332–8.
13. Ben Naftali Y, Duek OS, Rafaeli S, et al. Plastic surgery faces the web: analysis of the popular social media for plastic surgeons. Plast Reconstr Surg Glob Open 2018;6(12):e1958.
14. Chandawarkar AA, Gould DJ, Stevens GW. The top 100 social media influencers in plastic surgery on Twitter: who should you be following? Aesthet Surg J 2018;28(8):913–7.

The Best Business Moves You Can Use To Enhance Your Practice

Samuel M. Lam, MD, FISHRS

KEYWORDS

- Unique selling proposition • Videos • Leadership • Long tail • Business • Plastic surgery practice
- Gross margin • Internal sales

KEY POINTS

- Leadership is the key to running a successful practice, following the principles of John Maxwell. Leadership always begins at the top.
- It is important to have a well-defined understanding of a unique selling proposition (USP) and leverage long tail strategies to attract patients. Videos are one of the most important ways to spread the information about a USP to the world.
- Creating an integrated digital platform in the office can help cross-sell and upsell patients in an effective way.
- Focusing on internal product sales can be facilitated by streamlining stock-keeping units, creating private-label products, and striving for larger gross margins.

INTRODUCTION

Most surgeons lack practical business experience, and cosmetic/plastic surgeons own businesses that require constant attention, knowledge, creativity, and insight for them to grow in the setting of a competitive landscape that faces only further encroachment on a daily basis. Many practitioners who are tired of dealing with insurance and dwindling compensation enter the cosmetic market, often unskilled and untrained, to perform sophisticated procedures. These neophyte physicians combined with many who are well trained pose a threat to businesses, not to mention the rapid expansion of corporate medicine that has bigger budgets and savvier marketing campaigns. Despite these issues, a surgeon can easily master the arts of sales, leadership, marketing, and so forth. This article is not comprehensive in scope but offers a highly personalized, albeit biased, perspective on what has proved successful for my practice. It is my hope that even 1 or 2 pearls will shape success and enjoyment in a practice in ways that could not have been imagined.

LEADERSHIP, MANAGEMENT, AND CULTURE

I know the reader wants to dive deep into practical, actionable steps to improve a business. The most important element to success, however, does not lie in aggressive marketing, long work hours, or diversifying a cosmetic portfolio but instead centers on the principles of superior leadership and excellent culture. The 2 benchmarks that can be used to determine the success of these 2 principles are evaluating staff engagement and evaluating staff turnover. I have had staff with me 8, 10, 12, 14, and 16 years; and I have been in business for 17 years. I learned a lot about great leadership from my mentor, Edwin Williams III, who showed me what this is all about.

There is a great saying, "Employees join companies, but they leave managers." It is not the fault of the staff member who wants to quit; it often is

Private Practice, Lam Facial Plastics, 6101 Chapel Hill Boulevard, Suite 101, Plano, TX 75093, USA
E-mail address: drlam@lamfacialplastics.com
Twitter: @drlam (S.M.L.)

Facial Plast Surg Clin N Am 28 (2020) 523–529
https://doi.org/10.1016/j.fsc.2020.07.003
1064-7406/20/© 2020 Elsevier Inc. All rights reserved.

the fault of the business owner for either hiring poorly or for creating an environment that does not foster compassion, care, and growth.[1] Of course, sometimes staff must leave due to personal reasons or desires to enter a different field, but it is imperative that the leadership at the top sets the tone for a practice, to diminish the odds of this happening, because staff turnover is the costliest expense a company can incur. Often, poor leaders blame the staff, but leadership and culture always begin at the top, with the surgeon leading the team. The surgeon's integrity, passion, skills, and leadership will steadfastly grow and nurture the business and minimize the risk of losing valuable employees.

One of the key authors who has shaped my thinking on leadership is John Maxwell.[2,3] He says that a leader who is a 6 (of 10) can only hire individuals lower than a 6. If a leader is an 8 (of 10), that leader can hire up to a 7. These numbers do not refer to the intelligence of the leader, because leaders always should try to higher smarter people than they are. They mean that leaders should be at an 8 for leadership skills. People who are poor leaders have a hard time attracting talent, and talent does not stay. Leadership is about caring about staff; as Maxwell says, "no one cares about how much you know until they know how much you care." Leadership is about inspiring them to be better by showing them passion and integrity. If leaders behave unethically at home and at work, the staff will know it and that will break down morale. If leaders are unethical, they will not have staff below them who are ethical either. Ethical staff will not work for an unethical boss, at least not for long.

A leader also train must leaders, another Maxwellism. It is too hard, if not impossible, to have everyone follow 1 leader. I aspire to have multiple levels of leaders in my organization who can help lead new staff or junior staff. How is it known that someone is a leader? It is not by a title, but it is the natural gravitation that people have toward that person. A leader can be identified because other staff ask them questions and model their behavior after that person. It is a de facto leader not a de jure leader. That said, there must be a real chain of command at a facility or things break down. I had a senior staff member come to ask me a question and ask for permission to do something contrary to what she was told she could do by her superior. I told her I could not answer this question but that she must go through the chain of command. The reason is that it is like having 2 parents, where the child asks the more lenient parent for permission to do something and that undermines the other parent. There must be a respected chain of command and that hierarchy must be honored.

Another fact I have heard is that there is a natural tension between sales and operations. If there is not this tension, then either side is not doing its job. Sales always will want to push the envelope to close a sale and to drive profitability. Operations always will take precedence on safety and structure. I have seen this tension creep up many times and it is a careful dance to ensure that no egos are bruised and that patients are safely and effectively taken care of without losing sales.

One thing I observed with Ed Williams, my mentor, is that he absolutely never lost his cool. I like what he said to me, "You cannot control people if you cannot control yourself." I always saw him take responsibility for what was going on even if it clearly was not his fault. I never saw him get angry, and I have followed suit from this model. I believe that I have never raised my voice or lost my cool in front of my staff in 17 years of practice, and I suffered from serious anger issues in my 20s. Everyone can change, and it is important to begin working on self-improvement. A lot of times leaders are so worried about fixing a person or a staff member that, if they would just work on themselves toward greater leadership maturity, the problem often would fix itself or at least the person would trust the leader more to fix it.

Another maxim is, "hire slowly, fire quickly." Geoff Smart's book *Who* is amazing for teaching how to hire better and that, if someone does not work, to fire that person quickly.[4] Do not let the cancer grow. Hiring against weaknesses is what teamwork is all about. If every staff member is identical to the leader in every way, then a business will falter. If leaders think they are the best in certain ways and do not entertain or foster debate or criticism for what they are doing, however, they also endanger the success of the business. I can write pages more on the topic of leadership, but no one says it better than Maxwell. The *21 Irrefutable Laws of Leadership* and *Leadership Gold* are must-reads.[2,3]

UNIQUE SELLING PROPOSITIONS, LONG TAIL STRATEGIES, AND VIDEOS

This section is a hodgepodge of ideas that have worked for my business development, but there is some thematic unity in the topics. One of the most important elements in business that a physician can strive to achieve is a definable unique selling proposition (USP). Most often, a surgeon fails to define what makes a business different from a competitor. Ideally, a USP is so unique that the surgeon achieves a blue ocean strategy, in which there is almost no one else competing in the field.[5] If this idea cannot be articulated or the surgeon does not believe that they have a unique identity, it is time to sit down to think through what makes that surgeon different. It begins with a very large vision of where the surgeon wants to be in 1 year, 5 years, and 10 years, and it can be a mixture of personal and professional goals. The surgeon should sit down and do what I call a "hot pen" exercise, writing continuously in a free-form way without hesitation or a break for, say, 10 minutes to 20 minutes about where the surgeon envisions themself in 1 year, then do it again for 5-year goals, and then do it again for 10-year goals. This aerial view of where a surgeon would like to be, often an expression of subconscious desires, can help frame where the surgeon needs to be. Things that define my facial practice as USPs are as follows: an artist who personally performs the full gamut of nonsurgical and surgical enhancement for the facial plastic surgery patient, controlling the total patient experience and results, and who has a sensitivity to painless treatments and natural results that are gender, age, and ethnically appropriate. For my hair practice, it is to be a leader in the field of hair restoration who practices artistic and technical hair restoration in a painless way, covering the gamut of hair disease (eyebrows, female and male pattern hair loss, ethnic, corrective, scars, and so forth) surgically and non-surgically for men and women of all ethnicities using advanced regenerative medicine and only performing 1 surgery a day.

A related topic to the USP is the idea of the long tail strategy. This concept is taken from the book, *The Long Tail*,[6] that in summary talks about how in the age of the Internet people are searching for refined topics like "Iranian corrective eyebrow transplant after chemotherapy" and finding a surgeon who has experience in this field and who has sufficient before-and-after photographs to justify a flight to see that surgeon. I have truly tried to focus on USPs/long tails that other surgeons in my field do not perform: keloid excision, lip corrections, ethnic eyebrow hair transplant, and so forth. Finding a USP/long tail can help diversify a practice, and a higher margin can be charged for a procedure on which a surgeon is deemed an authority.

Now, how is this USP/long tail marketed? Videos! I have been uploading videos to YouTube.com since December 2006, long before it was even fashionable. To understand more in-depth how I use videos, just visit my channel *samlammd* and see what would work and what would not. For me, the single best type of video that has worked is filming myself when I am on podium at major scientific programs. I use a wireless microphone, a low-light video camera, and a portable tripod. Videos need to be authentic. I can write paragraphs on this subject but suffice it to say that they are the principal media by which I attract patients other than word of mouth.

SURROUNDING WITH BETTER PEERS

No matter how creative a surgeon is, it is far better to be surrounded with amazing colleagues and peers. I attend many scientific meetings each year and when I say attend, I mean I actually sit in the lectures and visit the exhibitors. I am looking for the most important pearl that can change my business. I talk with my colleagues in the hallway and ask them what has changed their practice. If a surgeon is not going to scientific meetings or are playing golf during most of the time, I would encourage rethinking this opportunity. I used to think that I wanted to lecture on podium throughout an entire meeting. Now I try to lecture as little as I can so that I can focus on learning. Lecturing too much disrupts my ability to focus on learning but I always want to continue to contribute so I still lecture (which I absolutely love to do), and, as discussed, it provides a wonderful marketing opportunity. I also gain a lot of experience and pearls through private Facebook groups with other facial plastic and plastic surgeons. Sharing private thoughts about new business opportunities with my colleagues has really helped build my business.

I have been part of a group called Entrepreneurs' Organization for well over a decade. To qualify, a member must own a business outside of just being a sole proprietor. I qualify with my owning a salon, skin care line, and wellness building. I attend a forum, a meeting every month that lasts 4 hours, with a group of individuals who are all business owners but are in different, noncompeting fields from mine. It has been a master of business administration crash course for me, and I believe it has been instrumental in making me a better businessperson and improving my business. If a business owner does not qualify for the Entrepreneur's Organization, there are many other similar opportunities like Vistage that can help owners surround themselves with business-minded peers to help structure, drive, and offer accountability for a business.

A DIGITAL WORK ENVIRONMENT TO IMPROVE SALES

I am very focused on internal sales. What I mean is that when a patient is already established in a practice, there is an ability to upsell and cross-sell them on many things. I have leveraged multiple digital platforms to be able to do this more effectively, upon which I enumerate.

From the moment a patients walk into my office, I have 2 large television screens that display my before-and-after images (**Fig. 1**). One screen shows only hair transplant before-and-after images; the other screen shows only facial plastic surgery and injectable before-and-after images. My staff email me a low-resolution screenshot of the before-and-after image. I then edit any color or lighting inconsistencies with my iPhone using the built-in photo editor. Then I use an app called Pixlr that crops the image to whatever format I prefer, usually 3:2 for most indications, 16:9 for YouTube, and at times 1:1 with the before image above the after image. Then I use a program called iWatermark+ (the yellow icon, not the blue version) to label the photo and/or watermark it (**Fig. 2**). I use these photos for my Web site and other platforms. In addition, I use a dedicated

Apple TV (third generation is sufficient, if a used one can be found) hooked up to the back of each TV. I create on my laptop 2 albums, "Face" and "Hair", and then, using my iPhone, I share the photo to the respective album and it becomes posted onto the screen. The Apple TV is set to random screen saver to show the images. The remote must be aimed to each Apple TV but away from the other Apple TV to set up the respective slideshows without interfering with the other one. It is important in my opinion to label the photo, "Rhinoplasty", for instance, because when the image flashes by fast, the label helps the patient focus attention on the facial area of importance.

Perhaps one of the best things I have done for my practice is acquiring the TouchMD platform for my office. Unfortunately, the company advocates using TouchMD to help with improving a consultation only and to send patients photos through their app. I wholeheartedly would disagree that these are the most important uses of this

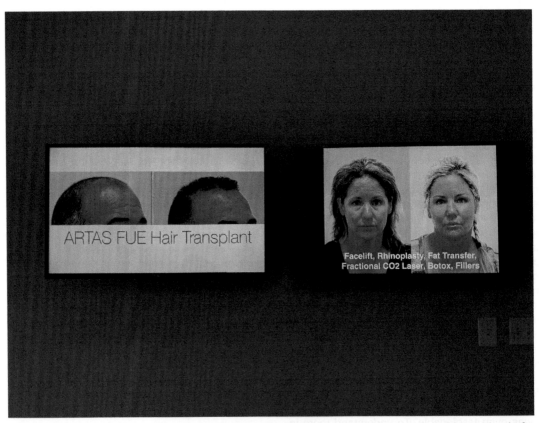

Fig. 1. This photograph shows 2 flat-screen televisions that face the reception area and display rotating before-and-after photographs. Each television is attached to a separate Apple TV: 1 television shows facial cosmetic surgery before-and-after photos (*right side*) and the other shows hair transplant before-and-after photos (*left side*). These televisions can provide reassurance to a patient who is waiting that the results that the surgeon achieves are natural and can serve as a platform for cross-selling a patient on other services that the doctor provides.

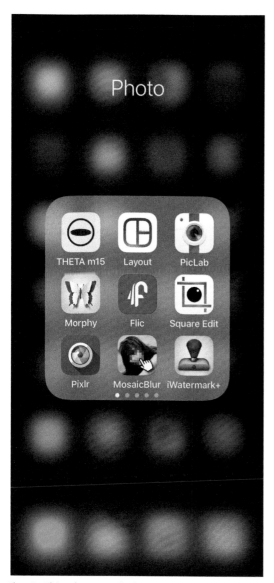

Fig. 2. This photograph features some of the apps used for editing photographs on the iPhone. In particular, Pixlr is used to crop and pair images, while iWatermark + can easily watermark and label the photos.

product. I do not even ask patients to download the app because I believe this is a waste of staff time. I use it specifically to cross-sell patients on other services while they are in my postoperative rooms. I use 27-inch Hewlett-Packard Pavilion touch screens in every room that have TouchMD built-in (**Fig. 3**). I can easily show a facelift patient my rhinoplasty results. I can scrub through a video of a laser recovery. I can show a magnified view of a facelift or rhinoplasty incision either in video or photo format. Every time I add a pertinent before-and-after image that I would like to

showcase, I e-mail it to my staff who then upload it into TouchMD. I also use it for consultations so that I can easily navigate between services I offer. I have divided the columns into Non-Surgical Face, Surgical Face, Non-Surgical Hair, and Surgical Hair. Simply put, it is the best cross-sell platform I have ever used. I also have shortcut links to my before-and-after images on my Web sites, to the homepages of my Web sites, and to my YouTube channel on the desktop of every computer in case a patient needs help navigating a particular part of the Web site and so forth. In addition, when the screen goes to screen saver, various products and services I am trying to promote appear on the screen and rotate every few seconds. I currently am working on incorporating short video messages into the screen savers

PRODUCT SALES

As discussed previously, I am focused in the office on internal sales. I believe one of the key elements to sales is also selling products, not just services. I am focused on a few things when looking at product sales: ease and speed of a sale, minimizing confusion with redundant product categories, large gross margins, and inability to the find the product online, for example, at Wal-Mart. I discuss each of these points more in detail to offer a practical strategy of how to create an effective product sales strategy.

In the past, I developed 4 stock-keeping units (SKUs) for my skin care line: an morning product, a night product, a a lighter version of the night product, and a cleanser. The problems are that (1) patients who are exiting the office after a treatment do not want to spend too much more money on products, (2) patients become confused with too many options, and (3) my staff has limited time to sell them a product. I changed my concept last year to reduce the product line to 2 SKUs: a single product good for morning and night and the same cleanser I had before (**Fig. 4**). Impulse buys typically are below $100 but I market my product at $165, which allows discounts for first-time users and for subscriptions. When I give my product on sale for $99, I definitely increase my sales quite a bit. I actually created and designed my own product that I am proud to sell. I have other products, however, that I have private-labeled with a company that gives me a much lower margin than the standard 100% markup. My own designed products afford me an 8-times to 10-times markup. The gross margin, defined as the product sale price minus the cost of goods sold, is a critical factor when I am deciding on products to sell. Having a

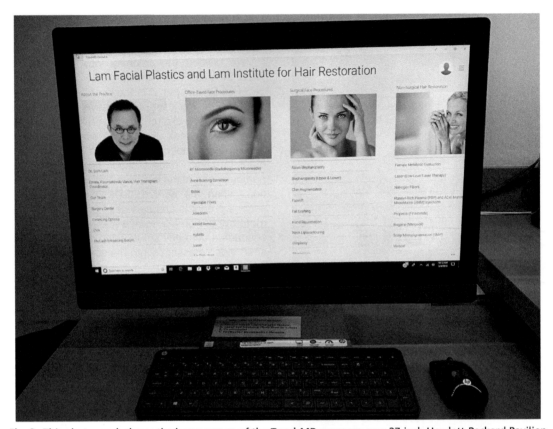

Fig. 3. This photograph shows the home screen of the TouchMD program on a 27-inch Hewlett-Packard Pavilion touch screen computer.

private-label product allows minimizing concern of a patient buying the product online and also allows having a more generous markup because the product does not exist elsewhere.

One of the biggest discoveries for me is Alibaba.com, where I can purchase products from China and have a 10-times markup with a low initial cost per item. For example, my hair fibers cost me $2.50 and I can sell the product at $32.50. The biggest expense of these products is the shipping, which in certain products that are heavy in weight can double the cost of the actual product. Because the margin is so favorable, this usually is still a negligible issue. Another problem is that the minimum order quantity (MOQ) often starts at 500 units but more typically is d1000 units to 5000 units. There also is a choice between original equipment manufacturing (OEM) and original design manufacturing (ODM). OEM signifies simply private labeling an already finished product; whereas ODM implies working with a company to formulate the ingredients of the product along with the container design. I have done both OEM and ODM. In most cases, OEM is sufficient. ODM is better if what a surgeon

if looking for cannot be found and the surgeon wants to develop their own product. Finally, a term with which business owners should be familiar is ex works, the base price of the product without the added cost of shipping, which, as discussed, can be high depending on the weight of the product.

Consumers can become confused with the plethora of products that can be sold to them. More confusion only leads to fewer sales. It is important in my opinion to streamline the portfolio to have as few SKUs as possible, especially to minimize or eliminate redundant items in a particular category. For example, carrying 5 types of sunblock can be costly and it can be difficult to sell ones that are less popular, especially if a surgeon plans to create their own or buy a large MOQ of a product. It is worth having a good spectrum of products, however, to cover different skin care needs: brightener, cleanser, moisturizer, shampoo (because I do hair transplants), and so forth. Again, looking at gross margins, MOQs, private labeling, redundancy, and SKUs all are important elements when developing a strategy for skin and hair care.

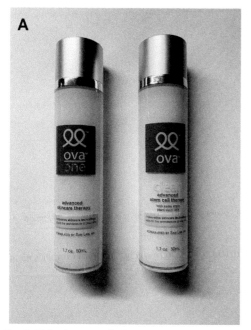
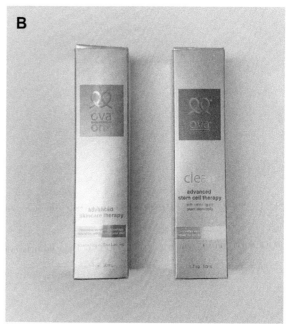

Fig. 4. This photograph shows the ODM products Ova One and Ova Clean (*A*) unboxed and (*B*) boxed that are a second-generation run of a private-label skin care line. The first-generation product had too many SKUs, were contained in breakable glass, were packaged in too large a box, and had too much liquid for travel. The larger format of the original product also made shipping costs unnecessarily more expensive, especially to protect the fragile glass. These errors were corrected in the reformulation of the product.

SUMMARY

The most important component of running a successful practice is superior leadership, which can facilitate hiring, retaining, and inspiring staff. Leadership begins with the physician who runs the practice and who must define the culture, lead by example, and cultivate staff engagement and growth. Often, physicians who run their practices do so in a vacuum without external support. Finding a peer network can be helpful provide feedback, accountability, and emotional support in the arduous journey of owning a cosmetic business. Physicians must have a lucid vision of where they want the business to be in 1 year, 5 years, and 10 years and be able to articulate a clear USP that may attract patients from across the world. Videos are one of the most powerful media to communicate the USP and should be authentic and diverse to capture the imagination of the public. Internal sales to patients can be enhanced through harnessing the power of digital media in the office through a variety of strategies outlined in this article. The physician should understand the intricacies of streamlining SKUs, private labeling, and gross margins when driving internal product sales. The business of cosmetic medicine is always challenging and changing, but physicians who are business owners can thrive when they fully embrace these elements as the impetus for growth and development.

DISCLOSURE

The author has nothing to disclose.

REFERENCES

1. Pink DH. Drive: the surprising truth about what motivates us. New York: Riverhead books; 2011.
2. Maxwell JC. The 21 irrefutable laws of leadership: follow them and people will follow you. New York: Harper Collins; 2007.
3. Maxwell JC. Leadership gold: lessons I've learned from a lifetime of leading. Nashville (TN): Thomas Nelson; 2008.
4. Smart G. Who. New York: Ballantine Books; 2008.
5. Kim WC, Mauborgne R. Blue ocean strategy, expanded edition: how to create uncontested market space and make the competition irrelevant. Boston: Harvard Business Review; 2015.
6. Anderson C. The long tail: why the future of business is selling less of more. New York: Hatchett Books; 2008.

Understanding and Getting Involved in the International Facial Plastic Surgery Community

Roxana Cobo, MD[a],*, Peter A. Adamson, OOnt, MD, FRCS, FACS[b]

KEYWORDS

- Facial plastic surgery • Otolaryngology-Head and Neck Surgery
- International Federation of Facial Plastic Surgery Societies
- International Board for Certification in Facial Plastic and Reconstructive Surgery

KEY POINTS

- The Internet revolution and creation of the World Wide Web in 1990 has ushered in an era of global sharing of medical information.
- Facial plastic surgeons are encouraged to participate in the outstanding educational programs being developed by the International Federation of Facial Plastic Surgery Societies.
- Facial plastic surgeons are encouraged to demonstrate their clinical excellence by becoming a Diplomate of the International Board for Certification in Facial Plastic and Reconstructive Surgery.
- Many international surgeons grapple with the issues surrounding the development or expansion of their own facial plastic and reconstructive surgery practices.
- Marketing and the importance of branding facial plastic surgery is stressed. The means to develop, and value of, a good reputation are emphasized.

INTRODUCTION

The Internet era and the creation of the World Wide Web in 1990 has ushered in one of the greatest revolutions in human history. In particular, it has enabled the sharing of information equitably around the world. This development has had an incredible impact in medicine, which doubles its data bank of information approximately every 18 months. English, not necessarily fairly, has become the international language of medicine. Today, practical knowledge of this language remains the only impediment to the acquisition of global medical knowledge.

As increasing numbers of medical professionals are learning and mastering English, they are not only increasing their own clinical expertise, but they are also contributing in a meaningful and admirable way to the advancement of medical knowledge. Internationally, the specialty of facial plastic and reconstructive surgery, borne of otolaryngology–head and neck surgery, and also practiced by colleagues in sister specialties, has benefited and thrived in this global environment.

The thrust of this article is to provide a deeper and better understanding of the development of facial plastic surgery in the international community. This explanation will, hopefully, encourage even more surgeons to become engaged and thereby strengthen our specialty organizations. The ongoing growth of the specialty, ultimately,

[a] Service of Otolaryngology, Centro Médico Imbanaco, Carrera 38A #5 A-100 cons. 222A, Cali 760042, Colombia; [b] Division of Facial Plastic and Reconstructive Surgery, Department of Otolaryngology–Head and Neck Surgery, University of Toronto Faculty of Medicine, Renaissance Plaza, 150 Bloor Street West, Suite M110, Toronto, Ontario M5S 2X9, Canada
* Corresponding author.
E-mail address: rcobo@imbanaco.com.co

Facial Plast Surg Clin N Am 28 (2020) 531–541
https://doi.org/10.1016/j.fsc.2020.07.004
1064-7406/20/© 2020 Elsevier Inc. All rights reserved.

facialplastic.theclinics.com

depends on this commitment from individual surgeons.

In addition, there are well-trained and skilled surgeons operating in the head and neck who may wish to enter or expand their practice into facial plastic and reconstructive surgery. Those who are younger or in more remote regions may not have had the opportunity to learn how to do so. This article offers some helpful guidance to build a successful practice and a satisfying career in facial plastic and reconstructive surgery.

It is hoped, and expected, that this deeper understanding of the origins of our specialty, combined with the acquisition of practical information to assist building a practice, will help to integrate our specialty. Individual surgeons will engage more with their local societies, and national societies will interact to strengthen the presence of facial plastic and reconstructive surgery on the global medical stage.

HOW TO BECOME AN INTERNATIONAL FACIAL PLASTIC SURGEON
Early History

Human beings have always had an interest in looking and feeling attractive no matter where they come from or how rich or poor they are. This impulse is reflected in the ancient history of humanity, where facial plastic surgery began as both a reconstructive and aesthetic specialty. Even though aging is not a disease, the changes that come with aging have always bothered men and women. Today aesthetic surgery is a multimillion-dollar business, not only in surgical fees, but also in cosmetic and minimally invasive procedures.

The practice of facial plastic procedures extends back thousands of years. One of the oldest surgical medical texts is documented in the Edwin Smith Papyrus, which is a transcription of medical texts from Ancient Egypt and date as far back as 3000 to 2500 BC.[1,2] In this text there is mention of a plastic repair of a broken nose.

Multiple other descriptions of facial plastic and reconstructive procedures have been documented over the years. What is interesting to mention is that procedures were documented, and that knowledge was transmitted. There are even reports of British surgeons spending time in India learning different rhinoplasty techniques and then traveling back to their countries to put in practice and expand their newly acquired knowledge.[3]

Specialists also date back to ancient Egypt and Rome, but did not really emerge until the nineteenth century in Western countries.[4] In the mid 1880s, specialties started to be recognized initially in France and Germany, followed by Great Britain, but it was not until the twentieth century that initial specialties were defined, boundaries between them created, and proper training of specialists instituted.[4]

First Otolaryngology, Then Facial Plastic Surgery

Otolaryngology is the oldest medical specialty in the United States that was officially created in 1903. Today, the specialty otolaryngology–head and neck surgery has 7 subspecialty areas. Facial plastic surgery, our subspecialty, is divided in 2 categories: cosmetic and reconstructive.[5] Although all otolaryngologists receive core training in these procedures, it became clear that, for those who wanted to focus exclusively in the area of facial plastic and reconstructive surgery, there was a need to create a formal subspecialty of facial plastic surgery and a society that could embrace all facial plastic surgeons. In 1964, the American Academy of Facial Plastic and Reconstructive Surgery (AAFPRS) was formally created.[6,7] In 1968, the first official fellowship training programs in facial plastic surgery began under the auspices of the AAFPRS.

Today, a facial plastic surgeon is defined as a surgeon who completes training in otolaryngology–head and neck surgery and then subspecializes in the treatment of defects of the head, face, and neck that are caused by congenital, traumatic, neoplastic, or aging processes. This specialist performs cosmetic and reconstructive procedures of the face, head, and neck, including minimally invasive and nonsurgical procedures.[8]

Facial plastic surgery has grown exponentially over the years and has evolved into an exciting specialty that encompasses 2 large areas: cosmetic and reconstructive. Additionally, the specialty today includes the development of nonsurgical minimally invasive procedures and use of energy induced technology (**Table 1**). Today, the field of facial plastic surgery has an overlap with many specialties, including plastic surgery, cosmetic surgery, oral and maxillofacial surgery, dermatology, and ophthalmology.

Facial Plastic Surgery Internationally

What then is happening around the world? Who is performing facial plastic surgical procedures? Is it also an overlapping field where many specialties contribute to the development of this area? How have other countries organized themselves to

Table 1
The field of facial plastic surgery

Surgical Procedures	Minimally Invasive Procedures
Cosmetic procedures	Neuromodulators (botulinum toxin)
Rhinoplasty	Fillers (absorbable, nonabsorbable)
Blepharoplasty, forehead lift, brow lift	Threads for Lifting (absorbable, nonabsorbable)
Facelift, neck lift	Microneedling
Otoplasty	Lasers
Chin augmentation, facial implants	Radiofrequency devices
Hair restoration	Chemical peels, dermabrasion, lipoinjection
Fat grafting	
Reconstructive procedures	
Facial fractures	
Functional rhinoplasty	
Local flaps, regional flaps, free flaps	
Microtia	
Cleft lip and palate	
Facial reanimation	
Craniomaxillofacial surgery	

develop the specialty of facial plastic surgery? Does it exist globally?

Even though initial reports of plastic and reconstructive procedures come from ancient Egypt, Rome, and India, international countries have been a lot slower in forming individual facial plastic surgery societies and specialties in this area. The European Academy of Facial Plastic Surgery was created as the Joseph Society in 1974 and finally became the European Academy of Facial Plastic Surgery in 1977. Its objective was not only to promote rhinoplasty, but also all other aspects of the specialty. In South America, the story has been similar. The first society created was the Mexican Society of Rhinology and Facial Surgery, which was founded in 1970, followed by the Colombian Society of Facial Plastic Surgery and Rhinology in 1983.[9,10] Today, countries like Brazil, Venezuela, and Ecuador also have facial plastic surgery societies.

For all of these international societies, the initial focus has been rhinoplasty. The reason for this has been the need to be able to perform not only functional, but also cosmetic, procedures on the nose without restrictions. Most of these societies have outgrown rhinoplasty and have progressed to the face and neck, many times changing their names completely or simply adding the term "facial plastic surgery" to their initial denomination.

In countries like China, cosmetic procedures and aesthetic medicine play an important role within its culture, and they have been working for a long time

in integrated care in this area.[11,12] The field of facial plastic surgery is now being widely promoted not only in China, but also in other Asian countries as demonstrated by the creation of the Taiwan Academy of Facial Plastic Surgery, the Pan Asia Academy of Facial Plastic Surgery, and the ASFAN Academy of Facial Plastic Surgery.[13] Despite all these efforts, it is important to note that most facial plastic surgery procedures performed in China and in other Asian countries are mainly done by plastic surgeons, except for rhinoplasty, which is also performed by otolaryngologists in some countries like Korea, Taiwan, and South East Asia. The only Asian country that has a facial plastic surgery society is Thailand (Written communication Dr. Yong Ju Jang). In Russia, the situation is not very different. Facial plastic surgery does not exist as a specialty. Plastic surgery was officially created as a specialty by the Russian Federation in 2009. Most facial plastic procedures are mainly done by plastic surgeons and some craniomaxillofacial surgeons, except for rhinoplasty, which is also performed by otolaryngologists (Written communication Dr. Irina Vasilenko, MD, PhD).

The International Federation of Facial Plastic Surgery Societies

Facial plastic surgery has grown and developed globally primarily because of leaders in the field who have shared their knowledge and taught what they knew all over the world. Once specialties were organized, the AAFPRS has been instrumental in the development of the specialty, not only in the United States, but also globally. This development would not have occurred had it not been for the vision and leadership of many American and international leaders whose interest was to promote and expand the knowledge of the specialty. This group of leaders, led by the AAFPRS, initially met in Washington, DC, in 1996 to discuss mechanisms to integrate the different facial plastic surgery societies that already existed. They foresaw correctly that this would stimulate and promote the growth and development of our specialty around the world. Developing their vision, they agreed to create the International Federation of Facial Plastic Surgery Societies (IFFPSS). In 1997, the first bylaws were ratified by the representatives of the founding member societies: AAFPRS, and the facial plastic surgery societies of Colombia, Mexico, Europe, Australasia and Canada. Today, the IFFPSS constitutes 13 societies of facial plastic surgery from around the world[14,15] (**Box 1**).

Box 1
IFFPSS Member Societies

American Academy of Facial Plastic and Reconstructive Surgery (Founding Society)

ASEAN Academy of Facial Plastic and Reconstructive Surgery

Australasian Academy of Facial Plastic Surgery (Founding Society)

Canadian Academy of Facial Plastic and Reconstructive Surgery (Founding Society)

Colombian Society of Facial Plastic Surgery and Rhinology (Founding Society)

Ecuadorian Society of Rhinology and Facial Surgery

European Academy of Facial Plastic Surgery (Founding Society)

Facial Reconstructive and Cosmetic Surgery (India) FRCS(I)

Pan Asia Academy of Facial Plastic and Reconstructive Surgery

Taiwan Academy of Facial Plastic and Reconstructive Surgery

The Brazilian Academy of Facial Plastic Surgery

The Korean Academy of Facial Plastic and Reconstructive Surgery

The Mexican Society of Rhinology and Facial Surgery (Founding Society)

Venezuelan Society of Rhinology and Facial Plastic Surgery

The educational mission of the IFFPSS

Educational meetings When the IFFPSS was established, it was clear that one of its main goals was to promote education in the field through congresses. The International Symposium that is organized by the AAFPRS today hosts many international speakers who come from the different countries who are part of the IFFPSS. These meetings are complemented by an international congress hosted by the IFFPSS every 2 years in different regions of the world. Congresses have been held in Mexico, Colombia, Italy, and Brazil, and the last meeting was held in Taiwan in February, 2020. The characteristic of these meetings has been not only the excellent quality of the academic presentations, but also that these meetings gather all people whose interest is facial plastic surgery. They have helped to promote the creation of new facial plastic surgery societies in countries where this area of expertise is just starting to be developed as a specialty. It has also become a valuable learning and productive networking opportunity for specialists from different countries of the world.

Archives of Facial Plastic Surgery The *Archives of Facial Plastic Surgery* has been the official journal of the AAFPRS and the IFFPSS since its creation. The publication has grown quickly and has become the preferred publication where many international specialists are able to publish their articles in the field. Its impact factor continues to grow, now being the third highest of 22 journals in plastic surgery. In 2020, the AAFPRS brought the journal in-house and renamed it Facial Plastic Surgery & Aesthetic Medicine.

International observership program The international observership program is a 1- to 3-month program offered so specialists can visit a selected specialist in facial plastic surgery in another area of the world. The objective is to stimulate interest in the field and complement areas of expertise from leaders in the specialty from around the world.

International fellowships in facial plastic surgery The International Fellowship Program of the IFFPSS is a newly created 1-year training program offered to specialists in otolaryngology and plastic surgery worldwide. It offers the opportunity to expand their knowledge and focus their expertise in the area of facial plastic and reconstructive surgery. The program follows similar guidelines to those established by the AAFPRS for their Fellowship Programs in the United States. The first accredited program was approved in Australia in 2018, and other IFFPSS country members are finalizing new programs that are pending approval.

This is a clear effort to elevate and expand the standards of the specialty globally. It is our hope that fellowships that already exist in international countries will embrace these standards to further enhance the practice of the specialty outside United States.

Certification and credentialing in facial plastic surgery: The International Board for Certification in Facial Plastic and Reconstructive Surgery The backbone of the IFFPSS has been its educational mission. Most countries do not have formal training programs in facial plastic surgery and many of the facial plastic surgery societies (except for the founding societies), are societies that are relatively young in their inception. In addition, as was mentioned elsewhere in this article, in many countries outside United States and Canada, most cosmetic procedures of the face, except for rhinoplasty, are performed by specialists other than otolaryngology–head and neck surgery and facial plastic surgeons. In 2004, after many discussions with the IFFPSS Board, an International Certification and Credentialing process was created. This established eligibility criteria using the American Board of Facial Plastic and Reconstructive Surgery examination as the final measurement of knowledge for all candidates. Even though it was an initial mandatory step, for many specialists it was not the board certification they needed or wanted. Finally, in 2012, 8 years later and after intense debate, the International Board for Certification in Facial Plastic and Reconstructive Surgery (IBCFPRS) was created. Today, 140 international specialists have completed all eligibility criteria, including passing a 2-day oral and written examination administered by the American Board of Facial Plastic and Reconstructive Surgery in Washington, DC. In addition, surgical cases are assessed, professionalism and an adherence to ethical standards are reviewed, and references are evaluated. With final approval, board certification and diplomate status are conferred. The interest in board certification has grown exponentially, and many specialists are looking for IBCFPRS credentialing to better enable them to practice, even in countries where the specialty or the respective society does not necessarily exist (**Table 2**).[13] Notwithstanding the valuable recognition provided by becoming a board-certified diplomate, the essential motivation for most surgeons who commit to sit for the examination is to demonstrate to themselves that they are the best that they can be as a facial plastic surgeon.

Impact of Globalization and Social Media on Facial Plastic Surgery

Globalization and social media are quickly changing the practice of facial plastic surgery around the globe. Most patients today use social media to receive information on possible surgical and

Table 2
Geographic distribution of IBCFPRS diplomates

Geographic Region	Number of Diplomates
Australasia	
Australia	7
New Zealand	2
South America	
Colombia	10
Brazil	5
Mexico	2
Chile	4
Ecuador	1
Middle Eastern Countries	
Iran	5
Israel	1
Saudi Arabia	1
Kuwait	1
Bahrain	1
Asia	
Hong Kong	9
Thailand	3
Singapore	3
South Korea	1
India	1
Africa	
South Africa	2
Europe	
Netherlands	23
Germany	12
UK	12
Turkey	11
Spain	5
Poland	3
Switzerland	4
Croatia	2
Belgium	3
Norway	2
Sweden	1
Portugal	1
Greece	1
Azerbaijan	1

nonsurgical procedures they could be interested in. The most frequently used platforms are Facebook, Instagram, Linked In, and Twitter. When patients come to our offices, a good percentage of them have already read about the procedures and have read about us as specialists.[16,17] There is a downside to this circumstance, because it is impossible to regulate what is published on social media, which in the end can lead to patients having unrealistic expectations. Additionally, patients constantly use platforms where chats are created, commenting on surgical procedures and on specialists as well. Today, it is impossible to regulate the content of these sites, and physicians have to be vigilant when they engage in conversations with patients on the web. Confidentiality issues must always be considered.

Word of mouth is still perhaps the most important patient referral system.[18] Patients use social media but, in the end, choose a specialist who has also been positively referred by another patient. This is more difficult for patients who travel abroad for surgery.

All this being said, what we are seeing today is that patients come to our offices asking for specific procedures. This huge input of information has expanded our specialty and, in many cases, has helped specialists to evolve from not only performing rhinoplasties, but to start exploring additional areas in our field.

How Can We Help to Stimulate the Growth of Facial Plastic Surgery Globally?

As mentioned elsewhere in this article, globalization and social media have catapulted awareness about facial plastic surgical procedures to the general public. Patients know more, and want more and we as specialists need to keep up the pace in a responsible and ethical manner.

Facial plastic surgery is a subspecialty of otolaryngology–head and neck surgery in United States and in some countries worldwide (eg, Colombia and others). It becomes important to make sure that all facial plastic cosmetic and reconstructive surgical procedures are included in the academic programs of our core specialties. A well-rounded otolaryngologist–head and neck surgeon should have had exposure during his or her training, not only to cosmetic and functional rhinoplasty. He or she should also have knowledge about trauma, facial reconstruction, and additional facial cosmetic procedures. This knowledge will increase awareness in this exciting field. Sharing knowledge, teaching, and learning from those who know more or are more experienced will definitely help develop our specialty globally.

Internationally, access to information is not always easy or inexpensive. How can we help specialists who are not formally trained in facial plastic surgery? Does this disqualify them from ever being able to develop their interest and skills? Will they never be able to perform facial plastic cosmetic and reconstructive procedures? A well-trained otolaryngologist–head and neck surgeon who has been exposed to all areas of the specialty should be able to perform most facial plastic and reconstructive procedures.

It then becomes important to facilitate access to information and, when possible, training in different areas of the specialty. Access to specialty journals has improved. The AAFPRS and the IFFPSS have the *Facial Plastic Surgery & Aesthetic Medicine* as a peer-reviewed journal where specialists from all countries of the world can publish their work in the field. Through the IFFPSS, mechanisms have been created to build bridges for those who want or need more exposure in the field. The Observership Program is a good way to start for those whose interest is facial plastic surgery.

The most recent project of the IFFPSS, the International Fellowship in Facial Plastic Surgery, will give leading facial plastic surgeons around the globe the opportunity to educate young specialists in our field. All programs will be constantly reviewed and supported by the Fellowship Committee of the IFFPSS, which is formed by specialists with experience in this area. This program is a 1-year program where, at its completion, all candidates are required to take the IBCFPRS examination in facial plastic surgery. Complete certification is obtained 2 years after completing a fellowship program and submitting a report of cases in which it can be amply demonstrated that the specialist is performing an adequate number of cosmetic and/or reconstructive cases in facial plastic surgery, as well as meeting other professional criteria. This will not only create new and more proficient surgeons, it will also enhance the professional life of the fellowship director.

HOW TO BUILD YOUR CAREER IN FACIAL PLASTIC SURGERY
The Plan

Whether a young surgeon decides in medical school, or a mid-career surgeon decides in midlife, to establish a practice in facial plastic and reconstructive surgery, many of the strategies to initiate and become successful remain the same.

Many have heard the aphorism of the 5 P's namely, prior planning prevents poor performance. Essential for any ultimately successful endeavor is planning to define goals and determine desired results. A very useful tool to assist in this regard is The Strategy Circle.[19]

Simply put, first, write down your goal, namely, "To establish a successful facial plastic and reconstructive surgery practice." Second, imagine what the results of this would look like for you. For example, career satisfaction, independence from insurance cases, having your own private office and clinic, increased financial independence, and so on. Write down everything that could evolve from your success, because this will confirm for you (or not) that this is what you wish to do.

With this done, then write down all of the obstacles to achieving this goal; after all, if there were no obstacles, you would already have achieved this goal. For each defined obstacle (such as not enough capital, office or clinic space needed, not recognized for doing facial plastic and reconstructive surgery), write down the various strategies that would help you to overcome these obstacles. This then becomes your game plan, and you can next establish a project planner, whereby you organize and prioritize your work to be done to reach your result. Importantly, you must put a timeline on your project, because "A goal without a timeline is just a slogan." Now you know what you want to do, and why, how, and when you are going to do it.

It is notable that the 2018 AAFPRS member survey determined that 71% of its members were doing 75% to 100% facial plastic and reconstructive surgery, 23% were doing 50% to 74% facial plastic and reconstructive surgery, and 7% were doing less than 50% facial plastic and reconstructive surgery.[20] The point is that the development of a facial plastic surgery practice reflects a continuum and does not happen overnight. Commitment to your plan, perseverance, and patience are required.

Knowledge and Skills: The Cornerstones of Success

The previous sections of this article identify the numerous opportunities offered by the international facial plastic surgical community to become an outstanding practitioner. Each surgeon has his or her own preferred ways to learn, but almost always a solid knowledge foundation begins by reading basic textbooks such as *Facial Plastic Surgery* by Ira Papel, *Facial Plastic and Reconstructive Surgery* by Hadlock et al, *Preparing for the ABFPRS Examinations* by Wong and colleagues, *Rhinoplasty, the Art and the Science* by E. Tardy, and *Structure Rhinoplasty: Lessons Learned in 30 Years* by D. Toriumi, amongst many others.[21–25]

Several of the traditional otolaryngology–head and neck surgery texts also have excellent articles in sections written by facial plastic surgeons. These include Cummings, Bailey, Papparella, and others.

Within our specialty, Facial Plastic Surgery and Aesthetic Medicine is the "go to" journal. The periodic journal, *Facial Plastic Surgery* published by Thieme covers defined topics in depth and is also an excellent resource. Obviously, there are many other fine journals and books as well, but these particular titles provide a focus for the aspiring facial plastic and reconstructive surgeon.

As surgeons, we all remain students throughout our lives. It can be said, "We never leave the University of Facial Plastic Surgery." Some students like to personally observe colleagues who are recognized experts in certain procedures. Such professional exchanges are usually very enjoyable experiences, but a business challenge in time away from practice. The AAFPRS has an outstanding collection of edited teaching video tapes, with voiceover, on all aspects of facial plastic and reconstructive surgery. The academy offers a special discounted price for international surgeons, providing an exceptional opportunity to learn fine procedural techniques from the masters in our field.

Attending courses, although taking time from practice and not inexpensive, becomes a mandatory part of one's development as a facial plastic and reconstructive surgeon. Major courses include the AAFPRS annual Advances in Rhinoplasty course, its Aging Face Course, and its Annual Meeting. Today, there are also international IFFPSS courses held biannually, alternating between the AAFPRS and IFFPSS. Many of the IFFPSS member societies also have annual meetings and courses, and have the added benefit of being closer to home for those who live in these regions. Besides learning about recent advances and controversies in our specialty, these meetings provide a wonderful and enjoyable opportunity to meet colleagues and expand one's professional and personal horizons.

Transitioning a Practice to Facial Plastic and Reconstructive Surgery

With a plan established, and ongoing education a significant component of your practice life, how do you "make it happen" in your practice? There are many components to realizing your dream. These include performing good work (first and foremost), building a good business, marketing, and establishing a good reputation that has others building your practice for you.

Performing good work

As mentioned, before embarking on minimally invasive and surgical procedures, book knowledge and video or observational technique knowledge are mandatory. As a trained otolaryngology–head and neck surgery or plastic surgeon, basic (or advanced in other areas) surgical skills will already have been mastered. You will have determined that facial plastic and reconstructive surgery is your unique ability, meaning that it is something that you are excellent at and passionate about.[19] You will have committed to your goal. You will be persevering despite adversity; it is never easy being a pioneer. You will be demonstrating patience, and you will be continuing to study and learn, getting a great sense of achievement and pride each step along your journey.

Ideally, a surgeon moves from an area or procedure of technical expertise to push the envelope into newer, uncharted territory for him or her, but not so much as to go through the envelope and have a serious complication. It is to be expected that there will be some minor, resolvable complications. They are an inherent component of every surgeon's experience. From each adverse outcome, one must reflect and learn so as to minimize the incidence of repetition. Wherever possible, it is best to move incrementally, and to learn from the positive feedback you get from successful outcomes. For example, one's first facelift should be a short flap, superficial musculoaponeurotic system–type lift, not a deep plane lift. Apply the "KISS" principle, "Keep It Simple, Stupid" and analyze your long-term outcomes.[26] For rhinoplasty, especially, this means not just 1-year outcomes, but 5 years and longer. Discuss cases with colleagues; chat groups have become a wonderful way to do this. Form study groups online. Join your regional IFFPSS society. Form an ongoing relationship with a mentor, and talk to him or her monthly. As soon as you are ready, prepare for the IBCFPRS examination, and pull together your cases to meet all of the requirements to become a Diplomate of the IBCFPRS (www.ibcfprs.org). This distinction will identify you as a surgeon who has met the highest standards and is a leader in our specialty. It will then become your turn to be a mentor for your younger colleagues who aspire to build what you have achieved.

Building a successful business

One of the first decisions to be made is how and where to practice. For example, in United States, about 45% of facial plastic and reconstructive surgeons are in solo practice, 38% in group practice (either as part of an otolaryngology–head and neck surgery group or with other facial plastic and reconstructive surgeons), and 16% are in academic practice.[20] The point is, there is no right or wrong; there is only the best choice for you. Being in private practice offers independence, but increased responsibility for outcome, and sometimes longer hours. Academic practices can offer more resident support and possibly research opportunities, sometimes shorter hours, but often less independence and a lower financial return. Group practices often fall in between these two. The types of procedures performed by AAFPRS surgeons are outlined in **Table 3** and **Table 5**, and the average numbers of each of these procedures is provided in **Tables 4** and **6**, describes the percentage of facial plastic and reconstructive surgery performing minimally invasive procedures, and **Table 6** the average number. It is to be expected that these procedures and numbers may vary significantly from country to country and surgeon to surgeon, depending upon their practice profile. However, they provide information that can help aspiring facial plastic and reconstructive surgeons know what real-world practice is like.

One of the best ways to build a solid business is to plan and manage using a tool called the front stage–back stage model.[19] This model is both a conceptual and practical framework to sharpen your organizational clarity. In essence, the front stage is everything you and your organization do to create value for your patients. The back stage is everything that occurs internally to support the value creation process.

You begin by identifying, in order, the various back stage methods that are required for a fully functioning business. For example, from marketing to telephone/email reception, to appointment management, to the consultation process, to

Table 3 Types of procedures performed by facial plastic surgeons	
Procedures	
Rhinoplasty	96%
Revision surgery	94%
Blepharoplasty	93%
Facelift	90%
Forehead lift	82%
Chin augmentation	74%
Facial implants	43%
Hair transplantation	18%

AAFPRS Member Survey 2018.

Table 4
Average number of procedures performed by a facial plastic surgeon

Procedures	Average Number
Rhinoplasty	72
Blepharoplasty	49
Revision surgery	47
Facelift	35
Chin augmentation	30
Facial implant	21
Forehead lift	13
Hair transplantation	2

AAFPRS Member Survey 2018.

Table 6
Average number minimally invasive procedures performed by FPS

Minimally Invasive Procedures	Average Number
Botox (myomodulators)	462
Fillers	332
Skin treatments	155
Platelet-rich plasma injections	41
Noninvasive fat reduction	22
Fat dissolving injections	25
Fat grafting	14

AAFPRS Member Survey 2018.

preoperative preparation, to clinic management, to accounting, to postoperative care, and to follow-up, and so on. There are many other, more refined steps that also need to be defined and detailed within this matrix. The goal of developing your back stage method is to create support for everything behind the scenes that creates and supports what is presented to your patients. It also is used to integrate the skills and improve teamwork among your staff. It continually increases coordination among all of your back stage methods. These back stage business activities represent your overhead, and constant application to improve your back stage method will result in increased productivity. This is the part of the business the patients do not see, just as they do not see the light, sound, and costume technicians or equipment that make up the back stage of a Broadway production.

Your back stage supports your front stage process. This is what your patients see and feel. This is what creates their experience with you, which is much different and more powerful than

your having just provided a service. People will pay for a unique experience (think Disney World, Tiffany's, the Four Seasons Resorts, etc.) because they perceive there is value provided to them. Therefore, the experience is created by packaging all the services that you provide your patients so that they are unique and differentiate you from others in your field. This includes everything from your web presence to telephone manners, to office decor, to information provided by your staff, to your consultation, very much to the procedural result, and to your follow-up care, and so on. Everything counts, and your goal is to continually improve each stage of what your patient sees, hears and feels during their experience with you. This creates value and increases your revenues, because patients will pay for a gratifying experience. Think of the joy and satisfaction you feel after the curtain goes down on an outstanding Broadway play.

Applying the back stage–front stage model creates appreciative patients who return time and again, as well as refer others. In a business sense, they become an annuity. The alternative is to attract patients on price, but this will not grow your practice with loyal and valued patients. Your practice becomes a hamster wheel. Remember, the patient who comes see you for a lower price will leave you as soon as he or she can get a lower price down the street. It becomes a race to the bottom as you and your practice become commoditized. This is an option, but for most practitioners leads to a less professionally satisfying career and burn out. There are no shortcuts to quality.

Table 5
Minimally invasive procedures performed by facial plastic surgeons

Minimally Invasive Procedures	
Botox (myomodulators)	98%
Fillers	96%
Skin treatments	80%
Fat grafting	54%
Fat dissolving injections	48%
Noninvasive fat reduction	32%
Platelet-rich plasma injections	32%

AAFPRS Member Survey 2018.

Marketing

One of the most important concepts to understand about marketing is that it is different from advertising. Marketing includes activities that promote or sell products or services, and includes market research and advertising. Advertising is a subset of marketing, referring to the production of advertisements for products or services. Good marketing adds value to your business, be this internal marketing within the practice or external outside the practice.

A major and critical issue in our specialty has been the branding of our name. Otolaryngology is an old and revered name but, unfortunately, in our connected world today only 3% of adults know what procedures an otolaryngologist performs (personal communication, Dr Peter Adamson, Decima Research Study, Canadian Academy of Facial Plastic and Reconstructive Surgery. Toronto, Canada, 1991). Only 23% of people think that an ENT doctor is even a surgeon, rather than a physician.[27] Ignoring this, some ENT doctors hope that potential patients will come to them for aesthetic surgery when, for all intents and purposes, no one recognizes an ENT doctor as one who does facial plastic surgery (other than functional rhinoplasty). In this day and age, these names are a losing marketing proposition.

Consider, in contrast, that 75% of the public thought that a "facial plastic surgeon" could do facial plastic surgery, almost the same as a "plastic surgeon" at 77%. Furthermore, it is notable that "reconstructive" surgeons are thought to have more training than "cosmetic" or "plastic" surgeons, and "cosmetic" surgery is thought to be less difficult and more temporary than "reconstructive" surgery.[28] Also, the media perpetuates the myth that "plastic" surgery is "cosmetic" surgery. In one study, 89% of articles used "plastic" in the context of "cosmetic,"[29] Keyword searches also show that "plastic" is used much more often than "cosmetic." The value of the brand name "facial plastic surgery" is virtually the same as "plastic surgery." If one wonders about the value of branding, consider Coca-Cola company has a market cap of $236 billion, assets of $90 billion, and a brand value of $73 billion in 2019 (Interbrand Global Brand, www.coca-cola company.com). In other words, Coca-Cola, the brand name, represents 81% of the company's asset value and 31% of its market cap (www.macrotrends.net).

To brand yourself as a facial plastic surgeon, understand your strengths, offer your patients a unique experience, become an expert surgeon, define your market, be value focused, and be committed to your front and back stage model. Having said this, always remember to spend more time on growing your clinical skills and improving your results than you do on marketing.

No amount of marketing can, in the long term, make up for poor patient outcomes.

For our specialty, Otolaryngology needs to become Head and Neck Surgery and cosmetic or aesthetic facial surgery should become Facial Plastic Surgery. All surgeons should use and brand these names, and our specialty societies should change their names to reflect the most positive branding possible. This is imperative in the electronic global village in which we live, where the first rule of survival is to be recognized.

Reputation

It is possible to achieve short-term success in anything, even with poor professional and ethical behavior. However, long-term, gratifying success is very elusive without a commitment to building one's reputation amongst colleagues and patients. A good reputation adds value to the worth of your practice; it is related to goodwill, which has monetary value. It is cumulative over time, is hard to build, and easy to lose.

Reputation can be defined as the belief or opinion others have of you and your practice. This is determined by a combination of your performance, your behavior, and your communication with others. Regarding performance, as surgeons we apply our clinical and surgical skills to attain a superb result, combining this with an exceptional patient care experience. This approach achieves the ultimate goal for the patient, the feeling that their outer appearance reflects their inner spirit. This outcome enhances their quality of life, confirming that they made the correct decision in selecting you as their surgeon.

Our reputational behavior is enhanced by always placing our patients' best interests above our own, and by always acting in a professional and ethical fashion. You, your staff, and your public relations people must all live by your message. This then must be clearly communicated, verbally by your staff, in all written and electronic communications, and throughout all social media interactions.

Today, rating sites and chat rooms provide valuable feedback as to your reputation. Although associated with many negative aspects, they can also be a useful tool to initiate reflection on your performance and behavior. They can help you to create clear and positive messages internally and externally.

And, finally, your reputation also depends on your integrity. You must always be truthful and live by your own values. All progress begins by telling the truth, and the first person you must be truthful to is yourself. By being honest with yourself and others about who you are and how you can best help others, you will make the most of your life as a facial plastic surgeon. In doing so, you will have much to celebrate, and leave an admirable legacy for others to emulate.

SUMMARY

Reaching out to the international community is not only teaching. There is much to learn from our peers from all over the world. Our minds must be open and we need to be able to accept change. To go a step further in the field, there must be passion for knowledge, recognizing knowledge is a 2-way street where, as we give, we also receive. By working together with our peers, we become stronger and we grow. If steps are taken in an organized fashion, with responsibility and ethical practices, our patients will be receiving the best from us. This will improve the quality of our specialty all over the globe. We should never be afraid of taking the necessary steps to move forward. We should, each and all, embrace our future. It is up to us. It is up to you.

REFERENCES

1. Mazzola RF, Mazzola IC. Plastic surgery: principles. Philadelphia: Elsevier Health Sciences; 2012. p. 11–12.
2. Shiffman M. Cosmetic surgery: art and techniques. Berlin (Germany): Springer; 2012. p. 20.
3. Stephen L, Last JM, George D, editors. The Oxford illustrated companion to medicine. 3rd edition. Oxford (NY): Oxford University Press; 2001. p. 651–2.
4. Weisz G. The Emergence of Medical Specialization in the Nineteenth Century. Bull Hist Med 2003;77: 536–75.
5. Available at: https://www.entnet.org/content/about-us. Accessed July 22, 2019.
6. Available at: https://www.aafprs.org/patient/about_us/h_fps_organizes.html. Accessed July 22, 2019.
7. Adamson PA, Gantous A. Once upon a rhinoplasty. The history of the "Queen" of Facial Plastic Surgery. Facial Plast Surg 2019;35(4):322–39.
8. Chuang J, Barnes C, Wong BJF. Overview of facial plastic surgery and current developments. Surg J (N Y) 2016;2(1):e17–28.
9. Available at: https://www.rinologiaycirugiaplasticafacial.org.mx/historial/ Accessed July 23, 2019.
10. Available at: https://www.cirugiaplasticafacial.org/ Accessed July 23, 2019.
11. Casas LA. Why should we foster core specialty collaboration in cosmetic medicine? Aesthet Surg J (N Y) 2013;33(1):171–3.
12. Feng L, Ouyang XP, Wang XY. Core specialty collaboration and integrated subject formation of cosmetic medicine. Aesthet Surg J 2014;34(2):328–30.
13. Available at: www.iffpss.org. Accessed July 25, 2019.
14. Cobo R. The International Federation of Facial Plastic Surgery Societies: promoting excellence in facial plastic surgery around the world. Arch Facial Plast Surg 2008;10(6):429–31.
15. Larrabee WF. The international federation of facial plastic surgery societies. JAMA Facial Plast Surg 2013;15(6):403–4.
16. Montemurro P, Porcnik A, Hedén P, et al. The influence of social media and easily accessible online information on the aesthetic plastic surgery practice: literature review and our own experience. Aesthetic Plast Surg 2015;39(2):270–7
17. Naftali Y, Duek OS, Rafaeli S, et al. Plastic surgery faces the web: analysis of the popular social media for plastic surgeons. Plast Reconstr Surg Glob Open 2018;6(12):e1958.
18. Janik P, Charytonowicz M, Szczyt M, et al. Internet and social media as a source of information about plastic surgery: comparison between public and private sector, a 2-center study. Plast Reconstr Surg Glob Open 2019;7(3):e2127.
19. Adamson PA. 10 tools to be a successful surgeon. In: Lee KJ, Chan I, editors. Essential paths to life after residency. San Diego (CA): Plural Publishing Inc; 2012. p. 415–26. Chapter 38.
20. AAFPRS 2018 Member Survey. Available at: www aafprs.org.
21. Papel I, Frodel J, Holt GR, et al. Facial plastic and reconstructive surgery. 4th edition. New York: Thieme Medical Publishers; 2016.
22. Cheney M, Hadlock T. Facial surgery: plastic and reconstructive. Boca Raton (FL): CRC Press; 2014.
23. Wong B, Arnold M, Boeckmann J. Facial plastic and reconstructive surgery: a comprehensive study guide. Switzerland: Springer International Publishing; 2016.
24. Tardy ME Jr. Rhinoplasty, the art and the science. Philadelphia: W.B. Saunders Co; 1997.
25. Toriumi D. Structure rhinoplasty: lessons learned in 30 years. Chicago: DMT Solutions; 2019.
26. Available at: https://en.wikipedia.org/wiki/KISS_principle Accessed September 29, 2019.
27. AAO-HNS survey. 2010.
28. Hamilton GS III, Carrithers JS, Karnell LH. Public perception of the terms "cosmetic," "plastic," and "reconstructive" surgery. Arch Facial Plast Surg 2004;6(5):315–20.
29. Reid AJ, Malone PSC. Plastic surgery and the press. J Plast Reconstr Aesthet Surg 2008;61(8):866–9.

UNITED STATES POSTAL SERVICE ®

Statement of Ownership, Management, and Circulation
(All Periodicals Publications Except Requester Publications)

1. Publication Title	2. Publication Number	3. Filing Date
FACIAL PLASTIC SURGERY CLINICS OF NORTH AMERICA	013 – 122	9/18/2020

4. Issue Frequency	5. Number of Issues Published Annually	6. Annual Subscription Price
FEB, MAY, AUG, NOV	4	$408.00

7. Complete Mailing Address of Known Office of Publication (Not printer) (Street, city, county, state, and ZIP+4®)

ELSEVIER INC.
230 Park Avenue, Suite 800
New York, NY 10169

Contact Person
Malathi SAmayan
Telephone (Include area code)
91-44-4299-4507

8. Complete Mailing Address of Headquarters or General Business Office of Publisher (Not printer)

ELSEVIER INC.
230 Park Avenue, Suite 800
New York, NY 10169

9. Full Names and Complete Mailing Addresses of Publisher, Editor, and Managing Editor (Do not leave blank)

Publisher (Name and complete mailing address)

Dolores Meloni, ELSEVIER INC.
1600 JOHN F KENNEDY BLVD. SUITE 1800
PHILADELPHIA, PA 19103-2899

Editor (Name and complete mailing address)

Stacy Eastman ELSEVIER INC.
1600 JOHN F KENNEDY BLVD. SUITE 1800
PHILADELPHIA, PA 19103-2899

Managing Editor (Name and complete mailing address)

PATRICK MANLEY, ELSEVIER INC.
1600 JOHN F KENNEDY BLVD. SUITE 1800
PHILADELPHIA, PA 19103-2899

10. Owner (Do not leave blank. If the publication is owned by a corporation, give the name and address of the corporation immediately followed by the names and addresses of all stockholders owning or holding 1 percent or more of the total amount of stock. If not owned by a corporation, give the names and addresses of the individual owners. If owned by a partnership or other unincorporated firm, give its name and address as well as those of each individual owner. If the publication is published by a nonprofit organization, give its name and address.)

Full Name	Complete Mailing Address
WHOLLY OWNED SUBSIDIARY OF REED/ELSEVIER, US HOLDINGS	1600 JOHN F KENNEDY BLVD., SUITE 1800 PHILADELPHIA, PA 19103-2899

11. Known Bondholders, Mortgagees, and Other Security Holders Owning or Holding 1 Percent or More of Total Amount of Bonds, Mortgages, or Other Securities. If none, check box ▶ ☐ None

Full Name	Complete Mailing Address
N/A	

12. Tax Status (For completion by nonprofit organizations authorized to mail at nonprofit rates) (Check one)
The purpose, function, and nonprofit status of this organization and the exempt status for federal income tax purposes:
☒ Has Not Changed During Preceding 12 Months
☐ Has Changed During Preceding 12 Months (Publisher must submit explanation of change with this statement)

PS Form **3526**, July 2014 (Page 1 of 4 (see instructions page 4)) PSN: 7530-01-000-9931 PRIVACY NOTICE: See our privacy policy on www.usps.com.

---

13. Publication Title			14. Issue Date for Circulation Data Below
FACIAL PLASTIC SURGERY CLINICS OF NORTH AMERICA			AUGUST 2020

15. Extent and Nature of Circulation			Average No. Copies Each Issue During Preceding 12 Months	No. Copies of Single Issue Published Nearest to Filing Date
a. Total Number of Copies (Net press run)			195	180
b. Paid Circulation (By Mail and Outside the Mail)	(1)	Mailed Outside-County Paid Subscriptions Stated on PS Form 3541 (Include paid distribution above nominal rate, advertiser's proof copies, and exchange copies)	126	116
	(2)	Mailed In-County Paid Subscriptions Stated on PS Form 3541 (Include paid distribution above nominal rate, advertiser's proof copies, and exchange copies)	0	0
	(3)	Paid Distribution Outside the Mails Including Sales Through Dealers and Carriers, Street Vendors, Counter Sales, and Other Paid Distribution Outside USPS®	20	16
	(4)	Paid Distribution by Other Classes of Mail Through the USPS (e.g. First-Class Mail®)	0	0
c. Total Paid Distribution (Sum of 15b (1), (2), (3), and (4))		▶	146	132
d. Free or Nominal Rate Distribution (By Mail and Outside the Mail)	(1)	Free or Nominal Rate Outside-County copies included on PS Form 3541	33	31
	(2)	Free or Nominal Rate In-County Copies included on PS Form 3541	0	0
	(3)	Free or Nominal Rate Copies Mailed at Other Classes Through the USPS (e.g. First-Class Mail)	0	0
	(4)	Free or Nominal Rate Distribution Outside the Mail (Carriers or other means)	0	0
e. Total Free or Nominal Rate Distribution (Sum of 15d (1), (2), (3) and (4))		▶	33	31
f. Total Distribution (Sum of 15c and 15e)		▶	179	163
g. Copies not Distributed (See Instructions to Publishers #4 (page #3))		▶	16	17
h. Total (Sum of 15f and g)		▶	195	180
i. Percent Paid (15c divided by 15f times 100)		▶	81.56%	80.98%

* If you are claiming electronic copies, go to line 16 on page 3. If you are not claiming electronic copies, skip to line 17 on page 3.

16. Electronic Copy Circulation		Average No. Copies Each Issue During Preceding 12 Months	No. Copies of Single Issue Published Nearest to Filing Date
a. Paid Electronic Copies	▶		
b. Total Paid Print Copies (Line 15c) + Paid Electronic Copies (Line 16a)	▶		
c. Total Print Distribution (Line 15f) + Paid Electronic Copies (Line 16a)	▶		
d. Percent Paid (Both Print & Electronic Copies) (16b divided by 16c x 100)	▶		

☒ I certify that 50% of all my distributed copies (electronic and print) are paid above a nominal price.

17. Publication of Statement of Ownership

☒ If the publication is a general publication, publication of this statement is required. Will be printed
in the NOVEMBER 2020 issue of this publication.   ☐ Publication not required.

18. Signature and Title of Editor, Publisher, Business Manager, or Owner		Date
Malathi Samayan - Distribution Controller	*Malathi Samayan*	9/18/2020

I certify that all information furnished on this form is true and complete. I understand that anyone who furnishes false or misleading information on this form or who omits material or information requested on the form may be subject to criminal sanctions (including fines and imprisonment) and/or civil sanctions (including civil penalties).

PS Form **3526**, July 2014 (Page 3 of 4)   PRIVACY NOTICE: See our privacy policy on www.usps.com

Moving?

Make sure your subscription moves with you!

To notify us of your new address, find your **Clinics Account Number** (located on your mailing label above your name), and contact customer service at:

Email: journalscustomerservice-usa@elsevier.com

800-654-2452 (subscribers in the U.S. & Canada)
314-447-8871 (subscribers outside of the U.S. & Canada)

Fax number: 314-447-8029

Elsevier Health Sciences Division
Subscription Customer Service
3251 Riverport Lane
Maryland Heights, MO 63043

Printed and bound by CPI Group (UK) Ltd, Croydon, CR0 4YY

08/05/2025

01864746-0014